Recent Advances in Endourology, 7

S. Naito, Y. Hirao, T. Terachi (Eds.)

Endourological Management of Urogenital Carcinoma

Recent Advances in Endourology, 7

S. Naito, Y. Hirao, T. Terachi (Eds.)

Endourological Management of Urogenital Carcinoma

With 58 Figures, Including 29 in Color

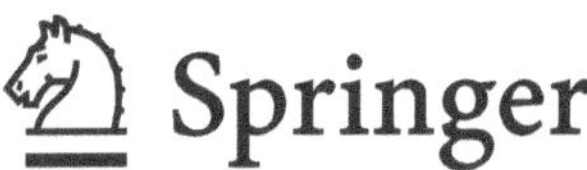

Seiji Naito, M.D., Ph.D.
Professor and Chairman
Department of Urology, Graduate School of Medical Sciences
Kyushu University
3-1-1 Maidashi, Higashi-ku, Fukuoka 812-8582, Japan

Yoshihiko Hirao, M.D., Ph.D.
Professor and Chairman
Department of Urology
Nara Medical University
840 Shijyocho, Kashihara, Nara 634-8522, Japan

Toshiro Terachi, M.D., Ph.D.
Professor and Chairman
Surgical Science Urology
Tokai University School of Medicine
Bohseidai, Isehara, Kanagawa 259-1193, Japan

Cover: Planes of neurovascular bundle dissection. *See* Fig. 5, p. 137.

ISBN-10 4-431-27785-4 Springer-Verlag Tokyo Berlin Heidelberg New York
ISBN-13 978-4-431-27785-9 Springer-Verlag Tokyo Berlin Heidelberg New York

Library of Congress Control Number: 2005932936

Printed on acid-free paper

Springer is a part of Springer Science+Business Media
springeronline.com

Typesetting: SNP Best-set Typesetter Ltd., Hong Kong
Printing and binding: Shinano Inc., Japan
SPIN: 11527602 series number 4130

Preface

The Japanese Society of Endourology and ESWL has published a monograph in the series Recent Advances in Endourology every year since 1999, at which time laparoscopic surgery had become popular, for not only benign but also malignant urological diseases. At that time, however, attention had been focused primarily on the techniques or minimal invasiveness of the surgery, and much of the data were still short-term. During the subsequent 6 years, long-term oncological or functional outcomes have been collected in various fields, and advances in surgical techniques and improved instrumentation have led to further, widespread development of such complex surgery as laparoscopic partial nephrectomy, radical cystectomy and urinary diversion, radical prostatectomy, and retroperitoneal lymph node dissection. Recently, the trend for laparoscopic surgery for small renal cancer has been shifting away from radical surgery to more organ-sparing procedures. Furthermore, recent advances in medical engineering have now made it possible to also use robotics for laparoscopic surgery, and new methods for laparoscopic surgery are continually being developed. Robotic assistance seems to be quite useful in performing laparoscopic radical prostatectomy and radical cystectomy with urinary diversion, both of which require an extremely high level of expertise.

While we have benefited greatly from the development of minimally invasive surgery, some serious complications have also been reported. As a result, the Endoscopic Surgical Skill Qualification System in Urological Laparoscopy was established by the Japanese Urological Association and the Japanese Society of Endourology and ESWL, and began being implemented in Japan in 2004. The skills of applicants were assessed by referees reviewing unedited videotapes of laparoscopic nephrectomies or adrenalectomies. In the first year, 136 of 205 applicants passed the assessment and were certified as laparoscopic surgeons with adequate skills to perform urologic laparoscopic surgery independently. This system is expected not only to improve laparoscopic surgeons' skills and reduce the number of serious complications but also to be a motivating factor for young urologists. Similar qualification systems may be established in other countries in the near future.

This seventh volume of Recent Advances in Endourology focuses on the treatment of urogenital malignancies with endourological procedures, including laparoscopic surgery with robotic assistance. The standard procedures and their relatively long-term outcomes or new techniques have been clearly described with detailed references. We editors are deeply grateful to the authors for contributing their educational and informative chapters. We hope that this monograph will be helpful in providing a better understanding of the present status of endourological management for urogenital carcinoma and, consequently, will set the stage for future improvements in both oncological and functional outcomes.

Seiji Naito, M.D., Ph.D.
Chief Editor

Contents

Part 3 Urinary Bladder

Part 4 Prostate

Part 5 Testis: Retroperitoneal Lymph Node

Contributors

Part 1
Kidney

Laparoscopic Radical Nephrectomy for Renal Cell Carcinoma

Yoshinari Ono[1], Ryohei Hattori[1], Momokazu Gotoh[1], Tsuneo Kinukawa[2], Shin Yamada[3], and Osamu Kamihira[4]

Summary. Laparoscopic radical nephrectomy has been developed and applied for patients with renal cell carcinoma since 1992. The number of patients undergoing laparoscopic radical nephrectomy has explosively increased worldwide in the recent years, and laparoscopy is extended to patients with advanced disease. It is very important to clarify the present status of laparoscopic radical nephrectomy among the treatment modalities for patients with renal cell carcinoma. Laparoscopic radical nephrectomy has a minimally invasive nature as well as long-term cancer control of patients with pT1–3a renal cell carcinoma comparable to open surgery. It is technically applicable for N1–2 disease and T3b disease if the tumor thrombus is within the renal vein. Also, it is feasible as cytoreductive surgery for patients with M1 disease. Laparoscopic radical nephrectomy is a standard treatment modality for T1–3a renal cell carcinoma patients. It is also available for treating patients with N1–2 disease, and for patients with M1 disease as cytoreductive surgery.

Keywords. Renal cell carcinoma, Laparoscopy, Retroperitoneoscopy, Radical nephrectomy

Introduction

There are various treatment modalities for patients with localized renal cell carcinomas available at the present time. Radical nephrectomy has been the standard therapeutic modality for patients with localized renal cell carcinoma since first being reported by Robson in 1963 [1]. Laparoscopic radical nephrectomy was first applied for patients with renal cell carcinoma in 1992 [2,3]. It has a

[1] Department of Urology, Nagoya University Graduate School of Medicine, 65 Tsurumai, Showa-ku, Nagoya 466-8550, Japan
[2] Department of Urology, Shakaihoken Chukyo Hospital, Nagoya, Japan
[3] Department of Urology, Okazaki Shimin Hospital, Okazaki, Japan
[4] Department of Urology, Komaki Shimin Hospital, Komaki, Japan

minimally invasive nature as well as providing cancer control comparable to open surgery. Laparoscopic radical nephrectomy has explosively increased worldwide in recent years, and about 10000 patients have already been treated over 10 years including 2500 patients in Japan. Laparoscopy is extended to patients with T3a and T3b (tumor thrombus in the renal vein) disease. As to small renal cell carcinoma, partial nephrectomy is sometimes applied even for the patient with normal renal function of the contralateral kidney, after Novic reported its efficacy in 1995 [4]. Laparoscopic partial nephrectomy has been developed and applied for clinical practice in recent years. Partial nephrectomy provides additional renal function of the residual diseased kidney but a risk of recurrent disease in the residual kidney [5,6].

Historical Aspects of Laparoscopic Radical Nephrectomy

Radical nephrectomy includes earlier ligation of the renal vessels before manipulating the tumor mass, an en bloc removal of the kidney and adrenal gland together with perirenal fatty tissue and Gerota's fascia, and dissection of the lymph nodes [1]. In 1992, we and Clayman et al. successfully performed radical nephrectomy by laparoscopy, in which the renal vessels were ligated after first identifying the ureter, cephalad dissection was made along the great vessels without manipulating the tumor, and the kidney was removed together with the adrenal gland, perirenal fatty tissue, and Gerota's fascia in an en bloc fashion [2,3,7]. The dissected specimens were removed intact through an additional 5- to 6-cm-long incision to make an accurate pathological diagnosis, and to avoid seeding of the tumor cell at the port sites and dissemination into the working space. The groups of Rassweiler, Coptcoat, and Matsuda performed this procedure in removing kidneys with renal cancer [8–10]. In these early experiences, the operative time was 5–8h, and the estimated blood loss was often over 500ml. However, the postoperative hospital stay and time to full convalescence were significantly shorter than those of the traditional open radical nephrectomy [2,10]. Laparoscopic radical nephrectomy has now been performed in more than 10000 patients worldwide and is regarded as a standard treatment modality for localized renal cell carcinoma.

Minimally Invasive Nature of Laparoscopic Radical Nephrectomy

Laparoscopic radical nephrectomy is appealing to the patient because of its minimally invasive nature. This is one reason for the worldwide increase in the number of patients undergoing such surgery. Laparoscopic radical nephrectomy was reported to have a minimally invasive nature even in the early experience [2,3,7–10]. McDougall and Clayman described in 1996 that an average dosage of postoperative analgesics was 24mg of parental morphine sulfate in 12 laparoscopy patients and 40 mg of morphine sulfate in 12 open surgery patients [3]. Time to full convalescence was 25 days in the laparoscopy group, which was significantly shorter than the 40 days for the open surgery group. In 1997, we also reported that a mean dosage of pentazocine was 34 mg in 25 laparoscopy patients and 63 mg in 17 open surgery patients ($P < 0.01$) [11]. Full convalescence was observed on the 23rd and 64th postoperative day, respectively ($P < 0.002$). Both studies clearly indicated that laparoscopic radical nephrectomy had a minimally invasive nature. Thereafter, similar results were reported worldwide.

Operative Methods of Laparoscopic Radical Nephrectomy

Certain technical issues exist in laparoscopic radical nephrectomy, i.e., transabdominal versus retroperitoneal approach, specimen removal (intact, fractionation, or morcellation), and lymph node dissection.

Transperitoneal vs Retroperitoneal Approach

In December 1993, Gaur reported a retroperitoneal approach for laparoscopic nephrectomy using a balloon dilator [12], which was subsequently used in radical nephrectomy [3,11]. We reported the clinical outcomes of 14 patients undergoing the retroperitoneal approach, and laparoscopic radical nephrectomy was a recommendable procedure for removing small renal cell carcinomas. The retroperitoneal approach should be considered for patients who have undergone previous abdominal surgery. Abbou et al. reported the results of 29 patients treated with retroperitoneoscopic radical nephrectomy in 1999 [13]. Laparoscopy patients had an average tumor size of 2.5 to 9 cm (average: 4 cm). Mean operative time was 2.4 h and mean blood loss was 100 ml. One patient required conversion to open surgery because of massive bleeding and another had colon injury requiring temporal colostomy (7%). Abbou et al. described that retroperitoneal laparoscopy is an alternative procedure in terms of technical aspect, morbidity, and operating time. While longer than for the open approach, retroperitoneal laparoscopy may be shorter than transperitoneal laparoscopy. Gill et al. also reported the results of 53 patients with localized renal cell carcinoma who underwent retroperitoneoscopic radical nephrectomy in 1999 [14]. Mean operative time was 3.6 h and mean blood loss was 225 ml. Two patients (4%) required conversion to open surgery and 9 (17%) had complications. Dissected specimens were removed intact through an additional incision. The mean postoperative hospital stay was 1.6 days. We, however, abandoned the retroperitoneal approach in laparoscopic radical nephrectomy in January 1997, and have used the transperitoneal approach in the most recent 213 patients except three with a history of severe abdominal surgery [15]. The retroperitoneal approach provided too small a working space for entrapping the dissected specimen into the laparoscopy sacks, which is necessary for fractionation or morcellation of the specimen and removal without an additional incision. Recently, Janetscheck's group reported that there was no difference in patient morbidity and technical difficulty for the surgeon between the transperitoneal and retroperitoneal approaches for laparoscopic radical nephrectomy in a prospective randomized study including 40 patients with Stage cT1 and cT2 disease [16]. Gill et al. and Abbou et al. use the retroperitoneal approach and intact removal through an additional incision. The retroperitoneal approach is preferred for patients with a history of severe abdominal surgery.

Removal of Dissected Specimen

The dissected specimen is entrapped in a laparoscopy sack in the working space and removed intact through an additional 6-cm-long incision, as described above. Any additional incision would compromise the less invasive nature of laparoscopy. To minimize the damage, Barrett et al. and Dunn et al. adopted a tissue morcellator for removal of the specimen without any incision, which provided the histology of the tumor, but not the pathological stage [17,18]. Another risk is tumor spillage from morcellation. Double-layered laparoscopy sacks are used for any damage by the morcellator. Barrett et al., however, reported that out of 85 patients no dissemination occurred in the working space except in one patient who had seeding of the tumor cell at the port site [19]. Rassweiler et al. has adopted fractionation of the specimens [20]. We also have used fractionation of the specimens since January 1997 for patients with less than a 5-cm diameter tumor where the tumor mass can be obtained intact [15,21]. Histopathological examination was possible on all 93 specimens and indicated six patients as having pathological T3a disease. In addition, no damage to the sacks was caused by scissors or the Kelly clamp. Neither seeding of the tumor cells at the port sites nor dissemination in the working space was found in the cases of fractionated specimen removal. On the other hand, Abbou et al., Gill et al., and Janetschek et al. still adopt the dissected specimens intact through an additional incision for a complete pathological examination [13,22,23]. We and Chan et al. also adopt intact removal for patients with large-sized tumors [24].

Lymph Node Dissection

In the treatment of renal cell carcinoma, lymphadenectomy has been reported to have no beneficial therapeutic effects. In its early stages the laparoscopic technique was too immature for dissecting the para-aortic lymph nodes, especially in right nephrectomy, which includes transection of the right lumbar veins and medial retraction of the inferior vena cava. We dissected the ipsilateral para-aortic lymph nodes in patients with 5-cm or more diameter renal cell carcinomas between 1996 and 2004 [15]. One of the 24 patients had micrometastatic lymph node disease. Extended lymph node dissection was able to be conducted safely by the laparoscopic procedure. Laparoscopy is now available for localized large-volume renal cell carcinomas, which may be associated with micrometastasis in the lymph nodes.

Operative Outcomes of Laparoscopic Radical Nephrectomy

Operative time was 3–5 h, including entrapment of dissected specimen and fractionation or morcellation. Abbou et al., Gill et al., and Janetschek et al. adopted intact removal of the dissected specimen through an additional incision with an operative time of 2.4–3.1 h [13,14,22,23]. Barrett et al. reported that the average operative time was 2.7 h, although they used morcellation [17]. Chan et al., Dunn et al., and we adopted morcellation or fractionation in a 5-h operative time [15,18,24]. Average estimated blood loss was 100–300 ml. Operative time was the same or longer with less blood loss when compared with open surgery. The rate of conversion to open surgery was 0%–8.5% due to vascular injury or injury to the viscera. The rate of complication was reported to be 8%–34%, with differences due to some authors including minor complications and others including major ones. Dunn et al. reported that the complication rate was 34%, which was lower than that of open surgery [18]. In our previous data, the complication rate of laparoscopy was 13%, which was higher than that of open surgery [21].

Long-Term Cancer Control of Laparoscopic Radical Nephrectomy

In 2002, Portis et al. reported the long-term outcome of 64 patients with localized renal cell carcinoma undergoing laparoscopic radical nephrectomy before November 1996 at three institutions including Washington University at St. Louis, USA, University of Saskatchewan at Saskatoon, Canada, and Nagoya University at Nagoya, Japan [25]. The control cohort consisted of 69 patients with localized disease undergoing open radical nephrectomy in the same period. The median follow-up was 54 months for laparoscopy and 69 months for open surgery patients. Five-year disease-free survival was 92% in laparoscopy patients and 91% in open surgery patients. Five-year overall survival was 81% and 89%, respectively. There were no significant differences between the laparoscopy group and open surgery group.

In our recent data, 316 patients were treated with laparoscopic radical nephrectomy and had pathologically proven renal cell carcinoma between July 1992 and September 2004 [26–28]. Thirty-one patients were excluded because they were maintained by hemodialysis and kidney transplants. Of the 285 patients, pathological stage was pT1aN0/NxM0 disease in 169 patients, pT1bN0M0 in 69, pT2N0M0 in 12, pT3aN0M0 in 14, pT3bN0M0 (tumor thrombus within the renal vein) in 5, pT4N0M0 in 2, and pT1–3N0–2M1 in 12. Two patients had lymph node disease and their pathological stage was pT1bN2M0 and pT3aN1M0 disease. As to long-term cancer control of patients with pT1 and 2 disease, the recurrence free rate was 97% at 5 years and 94% at 10 years in pT1aN0/Nx M0 patients (Fig. 1), 86% at 5 years in pT1bN0M0 patients (Fig. 2), and 70% at 5 years in pT2N0M0 patients (Fig. 3). The cancer-specific patient survival rate was 94% at 5 years and 88% at 10 years in pT1aN0/Nx M0 patients

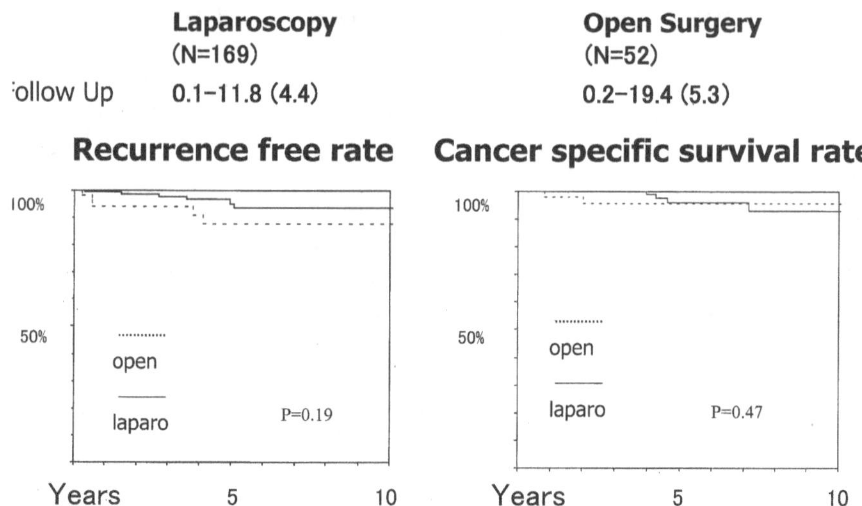

FIG. 1. Recurrence-free rate and cancer-specific survival rate in pT1aN0M0 patients who were treated with laparoscopic nephrectomy and open nephrectomy

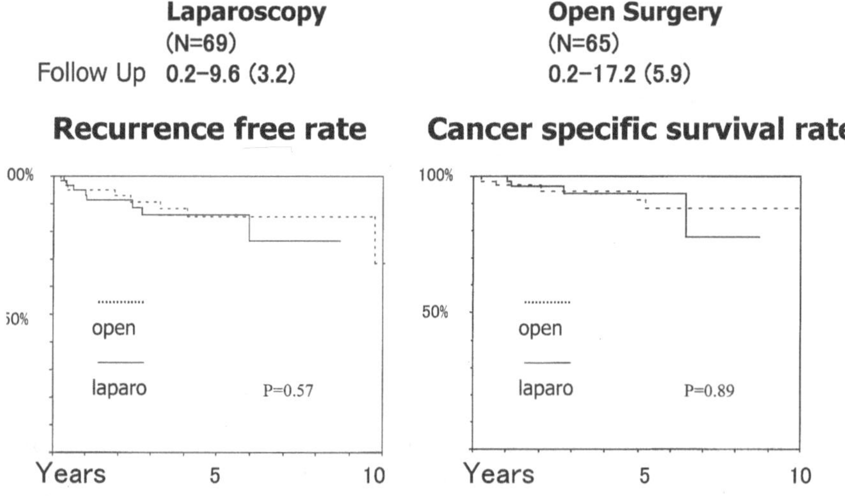

FIG. 2. Recurrence-free rate and cancer-specific survival rate in pT1bN0M0 patients who were treated with laparoscopic nephrectomy and open nephrectomy

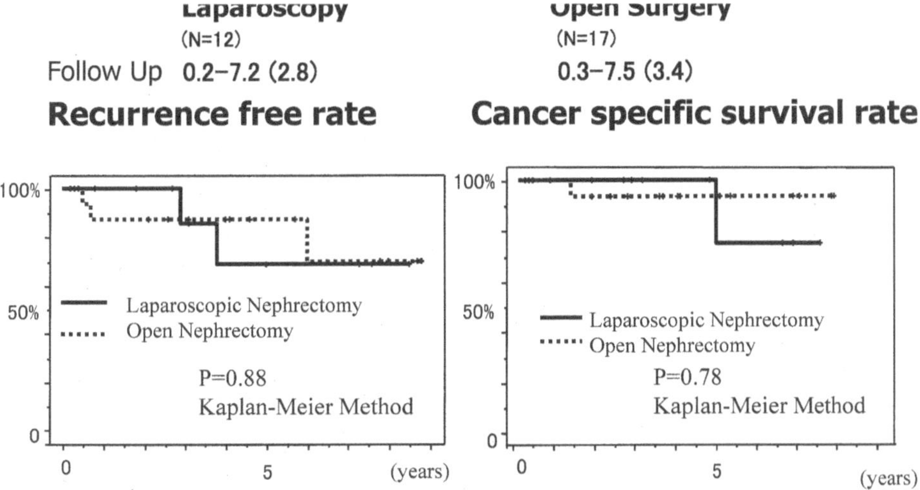

FIG. 3. Recurrence-free rate and cancer-specific survival rate in pT2N0M0 patients who were treated with laparoscopic nephrectomy and open nephrectomy

(Fig. 1), 86% at 5 years in pT1bN0M0 patients (Fig. 2), and 76% at 5 years in pT2N0M0 patients (Fig. 3). There were no significant differences between laparoscopy and open surgery patients. For patients with T1 and T2 disease, laparoscopy is available in terms of technical aspects and decreased morbidity. Laparoscopy is a standard treatment modality for patients with T1 and T2 renal cell carcinoma.

Laparoscopic Radical Nephrectomy for Advanced Disease

Laparoscopic radical nephrectomy is now applicable for the removal of the kidney in patients with advanced disease. Gill et al. described successful laparoscopy for removing kidneys from nine pT3a and 16 pT3b disease (tumor thrombus within the renal vein) patients [23,29]. In the pT3b disease, tumor size was 4.7–20 (mean: 10.1) cm. Of the 16 patients, 15 were successfully treated with laparoscopy and 1 required conversion to open surgery due to massive bleeding. Operative time was 1.3–5.5 (mean: 3.2) h and estimated blood loss was 30–1125 (mean: 374) ml. Wille et al. also reported a similar clinical outcome of 21 pT3a and seven pT3b disease patients who underwent laparoscopy [30]. We also had a similar experience involving 14 pT3aN0M0 patients, five pT3bN0M0, and two 2 pT4N0M0, as described above. Except for the two patients with pT4 disease, 19 patients were successfully treated with laparoscopy. Operative time was 2.9–5.6 (mean: 3.9) h and estimated blood loss was 10–900 (mean: 230) ml. Both pT4 patients required a conversion to open surgery for dissection from the

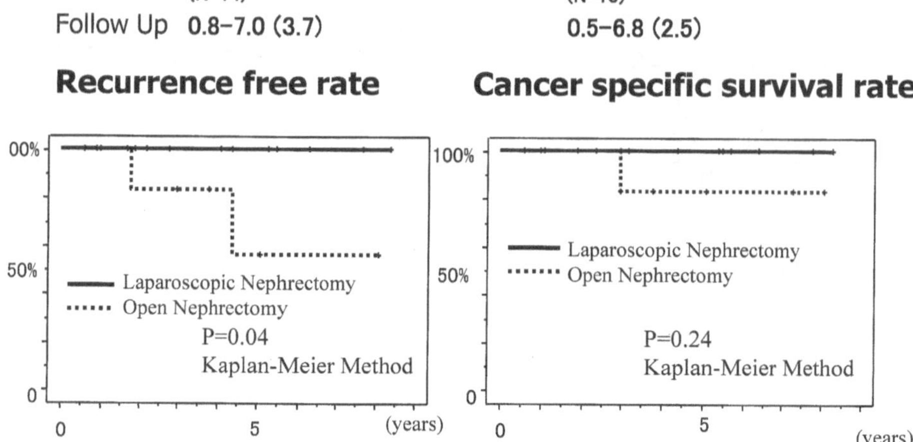

FIG. 4. Recurrence-free rate and cancer-specific survival rate in pT3aN0M0 patients who were treated with laparoscopic nephrectomy and open nephrectomy

psoas muscle and the colon. The 5-year disease-free and overall survival rates were 100% and 100% in pT3aN0M0 patients (Fig. 4). Of the five pT3bN0M0 patients, three are alive without metastasis 18–36 months after surgery. One had recurrent disease 15 months after surgery, and another died of other causes after 12 months. One pT4 patient died of cancer 8 months after surgery, and another is alive with recurrent disease at 33 months.

Regarding laparoscopic cytoreductive nephrectomy for metastatic disease, in 1999 Walther et al. reported its feasibility for patients with metastatic disease, although patients with T3b and T4 disease and massive lymph node disease were excluded from the study [31]. Of 11 patients, seven were successfully treated with transperitoneal laparoscopy and morcellation technique or intact removal. Laparoscopy was converted to open surgery in four patients. The tumor volume was 161–734 (mean: 443) ml and the diameter was 8–13 (mean: 11.3) cm. Mean operative time was 8.5 h and mean estimated blood loss was 1333 ml. Mean time to interleukin-2 treatment was 40 days. Walther et al. concluded that laparoscopy had beneficial effects on the patient requiring interleukin-2 treatment after laparoscopy. Mosharafa et al. also described similar results in seven patients with metastatic disease who underwent laparoscopy in 2003 [32]. We also had some experience with cytoreductive laparoscopic nephrectomy for 12 patients with metastatic disease; the tumor volume was 266–956 (mean: 523) ml and the diameter was 4–12 (mean: 7.9) cm [27,28]. Eleven patients were successfully treated with laparoscopy. Operative time was 3.6–6.7 (mean: 4.9) h and estimated blood loss was 50–2000 (mean: 435) ml. One patient had vascular injury, which was repaired by open surgery. Time to alpha-interferon therapy was 8–10 (mean: 8.3) days. The 3-year survival rate was 40% (Fig. 5). These data indicated that laparo-

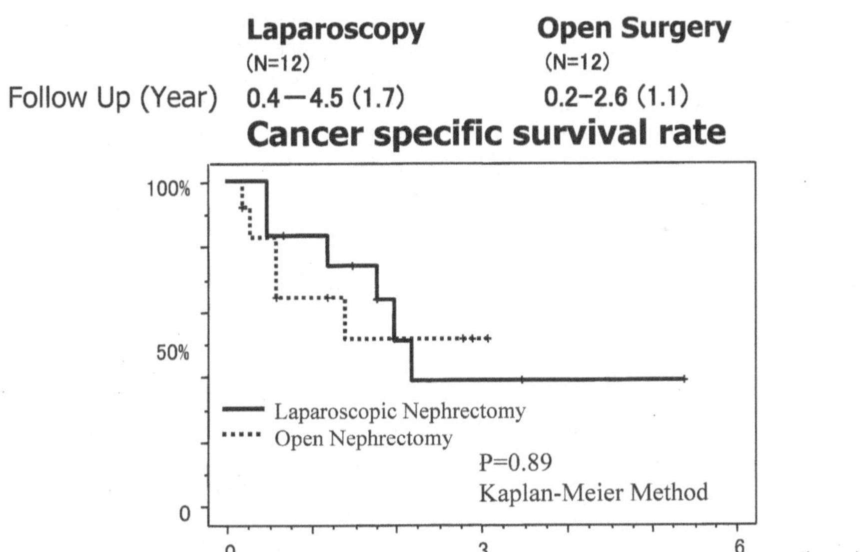

Fig. 5. Cancer-specific survival rate in M1 patients who were treated with laparoscopic nephrectomy and open nephrectomy

scopic radical nephrectomy was also available as cytoreductive surgery and provided early immunotherapy for patients with metastatic disease.

Conclusion

Laparoscopic radical nephrectomy has been performed in over 10000 patients with renal cell carcinoma worldwide. The dramatic increase in laparoscopic radical nephrectomy is due in part to the many patients who have benefited from this technology, with less pain and earlier recovery to full convalescence and normal activity. Long-term cancer control of laparoscopic radical nephrectomy is similar to that of open surgery. It is a standard treatment modality for patients with T1 to T3a renal cell carcinoma. In addition, it is available for selected patients with advanced disease. However, the development of safe and reliable techniques in laparoscopy is necessary for large tumors and advanced disease as well as the evaluation of cancer control.

References

1. Robson CJ (1963) Radical nephrectomy for renal cell carcinoma. J Urol 89:37–42
2. Ono Y, Sahashi M, Yamada S, Ohshima S (1993) Laparoscopic nephrectomy without morcellation for renal cell carcinoma: report of initial 2 cases. J Urol 150:1222–1224

3. McDougall EM, Clayman RV, Elashry OM (1996) Laparoscopic radical nephrectomy for renal tumor: The Washington University experience. J Urol 155:1180–1185
4. Novick AC (1995) Partial nephrectomy for renal cell carcinoma. Urology 46:149–152
5. Lerner SE, Hawkins CA, Blute ML, Grabner A, Wollan PC, Eickholt JT, Zincke H (2002) Disease outcome in patients with low stage renal cell carcinoma treated with nephron sparing or radical surgery. J Urol 167:884–889
6. Fergany AF, Hafez KS, Novick AC (2000) Long-term results of nephron sparing surgery for localized renal cell carcinoma: 10-year follow-up. J Urol 163:442–445
7. Ono Y, Katoh N, Kinukawa T, Sahashi M, Ohshima S (1994) Laparoscopic nephrectomy, radical nephrectomy and adrenalectomy: Nagoya experience. J Urol 152:1962–1966
8. Matsuda T, Terachi T, Mikami O, Komatz Y, Yoshida O (1993) Laparoscopic nephrectomy with lymphadenectomy for renal cell carcinoma: initial two cases. Min Invas Ther 2:221–226
9. Coptcoat M, Joyce A, Rassweiler J, Ropert R (1992) Laparoscopic nephrectomy: the Kings clinical experience. J Urol 147 part 2:433A, abstract 881
10. Tschada RK, Rassweiler JJ, Schmeller N, Theodorakis J (1995) Laparoscopic tumor nephrectomy-the German experiences. J Urol 153 part2:479A, abstract 1003
11. Ono Y, Katoh N, Kinukawa T, Matsuura O, Ohshima S (1997) Laparoscopic radical nephrectomy: the Nagoya experience. J Urol 158:719–723
12. Gaur DD (1992) Laparoscopic operative retroperitoneoscopy: use of a new device. J Urol 148:1137–1139
13. Abbou CC, Cicco A, Gasman D, Hoznek A, Antiphon P, Chopin DK, Salomon L (1999) Retroperitoneal laparoscopic versus open radical nephrectomy. J Urol 161:1776–1780
14. Gill IS, Schweizer D, Hobart G, Sung GT, Klein EA, Novick AC (1999) Retroperitoneal laparoscopic radical nephrectomy: the Cleveland clinic experience. J Urol 163:1665–1670
15. Ono Y, Kinukawa T, Hattori R, Yamada S, Nishiyama N, Mizutani K, Ohshima S (1999) Laparoscopic radical nephrectomy for renal cell carcinoma: a five-year experience. Urology 53:280–286
16. Nambirajana T, Jeschke S, Al-Zahrani H, Vrabec G, Leeb K, Janetschek G (2004) Prospective, randomized controlled study: Transperitoneal laparoscopic versus retroperitoneoscopic radical nephrectomy. Urology 64:919–924
17. Barrett PH, Fentie DD, Taranger LA (1998) Laparoscopic radical nephrectomy with morcellation for renal cell carcinoma: the Saskatoon experience. Urology 52:23–28
18. Dunn MD, Portis AJ, Shalhav AL, Elbahnasy AM, Heidorn C, McDougall EM, Clayman RV (2000) Laparoscopic versus open radical nephrectomy: a 9-year experience. J Urol 164:1153–1159
19. Barrett PH, Fentie DD (1999) Longer follow-up for laparoscopic radical nephrectomy with morcellation for renal cell carcinoma. J Endourol 13 suppl 1:A62, abstract PS4-4
20. Rassweiler JJ, Henkel TO, Stoch C, Greschner M, Becker P, Preminger GM, Schulman CC, Frede T, Alken P (1994) Retroperitoneal laparoscopic nephrectomy and other procedures in the upper pertoperitoneum using a balloon dissection technique. Eur Urol 25:229–236
21. Ono Y, Kinukawa T, Hattori R, Gotoh M, Kamihira O, Ohshima S (2001) The long-term outcome of laparoscopic radical nephrectomy for small renal cell carcinoma. J Urol 165:1867–1870

22. Janetschek G, Jeschke K, Peschel R, Strohmeyer D, Henning K, Bartsch G (2000) Laparoscopic surgery for stage T1 renal cell carcinoma: radical and wedge resection. Eur Urol 38:131–138
23. Gill IS, Meraney AM, Schweizer DK, Savage SS, Hobart MG, Sung GT, Nelson D, Novick AC (2001) Laparoscopic radical nephrectomy in 100 patients: a single center experience from the united states. Cancer 92:1843–1855
24. Chan DY, Cadeddu JA, Jarrett TW, Marshall FF, Kavoussi LR (2001) Laparoscopic radical nephrectomy: cancer control for renal cell carcinoma. J Urol 166:2095–2100
25. Portis AJ, Yan Y, Landman J, Chen C, Barrett PH, Fentie DD, Ono Y, McDougall EM, Clayman RV (2002) Long-term follow-up after laparoscopic radical nephrectomy. J Urol 167:1257–1262
26. Saika T, Ono Y, Hattori R, Gotoh M, Kamihira O, Yoshikawa Y, Yoshino Y, Ohshima S (2003) Long-term outcome of laparoscopic radical nephrectomy for pathologic T1 renal cell carcinoma. Urology 62:1018–1023
27. Kamihira O, Ono Y, Kinukawa T, Hattori R, Gotoh M, Yamada S, Ohshima S (2004) Long-term cancer control of laparoscopic radical nephrectomy for renal cell carcinoma. J Urol 171:338, abstract 1285
28. Ono Y: Laparoscopic radical nephrectomy. In: Higashihara E, Naitoh S, Matsuda T (eds) (2004) New challenges in laparoscopic urologic surgery. Recent advances in endourology 5. Springer, Berlin Heidelberg New York Tokyo, pp 11–23
29. Desai MM, Gill IS, Ramani AP, Matin SF, Kaouk JH, Campero JM (2003) Laparoscopic radical nephrectomy for cancer with level 1 renal vein involvement. J Urol 169:487–491
30. Wille AH, Roigas JR, Deger S, Tullmann M, Turk I, Loening SA (2004) Laparoscopic radical nephrectomy: techniques, results and oncological outcome in 125 consecutive cases Eur Urol 45:483–489
31. Walther MM, Lyne JC, Libutti SK, Linehan WM (1999) Laparoscopic cytoreductive nephrectomy as preparation for administration of systemic interleukin-2 in the treatment of metastatic renal cell carcinoma: a pilot study. Urology 53:496–501
32. Mosharafa, A, Koch M, Shalhave A, Gardner T, Logan T, Bihrle R, Forster R (2003) Nephrectomy for metastatic renal cell carcinoma: Indiana University experience Urology 62:636–640

Laparoscopic Partial Nephrectomy

James F. Borin and Ralph V. Clayman

Summary. Partial nephrectomy is emerging as the standard of care for small exophytic renal tumors <4 cm regardless of renal function status. In comparison to radical nephrectomy, studies have demonstrated equivalent oncologic control and decreased risk of renal insufficiency. While laparoscopic radical nephrectomy has been widely adopted as the procedure of choice for large renal masses, laparoscopic partial nephrectomy (LPN) requires a higher level of expertise. However, recent advances in technology, instrument design, and greater facility with laparoscopy among urologists have made this procedure more accessible. There is little long-term follow-up, but some recent large series demonstrate positive margins <3% and local recurrence <5%, commensurate with the open procedure. A transperitoneal approach is often used for anterior and polar tumors and a retroperitoneal approach for posterior and posterolateral lesions; however, if hilar control is felt to be needed, then a transperitoneal approach is usually used regardless of the lesion's location. In addition to standard laparoscopy, a hand-assisted approach can be used to facilitate suturing during renal reconstruction. Warm ischemia, up to 30 min, is usually necessary for large, complex, or centrally located tumors. When longer periods of warm ischemia are anticipated, cold ischemia may be employed via surface, transureteral, or intra-arterial cooling. Advances in surgical sealants continue to facilitate hemostasis; these include glues as well as hemostatic agents.

Keywords. Laparoscopy, Partial nephrectomy, Kidney, Renal cell carcinoma, Minimally invasive surgery

---

Department of Urology, University of California Irvine Medical Center, 101 The City Drive, Building 55, 3rd Floor, Orange, CA 92868, USA

Introduction

Renal tumors of epithelial origin account for approximately 4% of solid neoplasms. Of note, there has been a near doubling in renal cell carcinoma (RCC) rates over 20 years, from 2.3% in 1975 to 4.3% in 1995 [1]. The reason for this is only partly due to an increase in incidental detection [2].

Radical nephrectomy remains the gold standard for curative resection of localized renal cell carcinoma. Since the era of laparoscopic renal surgery was ushered in 15 years ago [3,4], the management of large renal masses by laparoscopic radical nephrectomy has evolved into the standard of care in most medical centers [5]. At the same time, there has been a paradigm shift toward nephron sparing surgery for small tumors (<4 cm), even in the presence of a normal contralateral kidney [6]. A combination of better imaging and earlier detection has resulted in stage migration for RCC, with a 32% decrease in mean tumor size [7]. With improved surgical techniques and historically good results for cancer control in nonelective cases, many urologists have questioned the necessity of a radical nephrectomy in the face of a small renal lesion. Retrospective studies from large-volume centers, such as the Cleveland Clinic, Mayo Clinic, and Memorial-Sloan Kettering, comparing outcomes of open radical nephrectomy with open nephron-sparing surgery, have concluded that both approaches provide equally effective treatment for patients with a solitary, small (<4 cm), localized renal lesion; cancer-specific survival is 89%–96% at 5 years [7–9]. In addition, McKiernan and colleagues retrospectively compared a group of similarly matched patients who underwent radical nephrectomy and elective nephron-sparing surgery and demonstrated a statistically significant advantage for the latter in freedom from progression to renal insufficiency [10]. At 10 years, Lau et al. found a significantly greater incidence of renal insufficiency, defined as an increase in serum creatinine to >2.0 mg/dl, in patients who underwent radical nephrectomy vs nephron-sparing surgery (22% vs 12%) [11]. In both studies, there was no significant difference in cancer-free survival between the groups. However, the incidence of recurrent or new disease in the renal remnant was 5.4% in the partial nephrectomy group and only 0.8% in the total nephrectomy group, indicating the need for more vigilant surveillance in the partial nephrectomy patients. Table 1 lists ten studies from the past decade [12–19] that document outcomes for open partial nephrectomy in 1405 patients. Disease-specific survival ranged from 88% to 98% and local recurrence from 0% to 7.3%, with a mean follow-up of almost 5 years.

Transperitioneal laparoscopic partial nephrectomy was initially described in 1993 for benign disease [20,21], but was shortly thereafter applied to renal cell cancer [22]; the retroperitoneal approach soon followed [23]. The widespread adoption of laparoscopic nephron-sparing surgery, however, has been relatively slow in comparison to laparoscopic radical nephrectomy. As such, much of the data are short term (see Table 2 [24–33]). Rassweiler et al. compiled data from four European centers for the period 1994–2000 [24]. In 53 patients there were

TABLE 1. Survival and recurrence after open partial nephrectomy

First author [Ref.]	No. of patients	Disease-specific survival (%)	Local recurrence (%)	Mean follow-up (months)
Moll [12]	152	98	1.4	35
Steinbach [13]	121	90	4.1	47
D'Armiento [14]	19	95	0.0	70
Hafez [15]	485	92	3.2	47
Barbalias [16]	41	97.5	7.3	59
Belldegrun [17]	146	91	2.7	57
Herr [18]	70	97	1.5	120
Fergany [19]	107	88	4.0	70
Lee [7]	79	95	0.0	40
Lerner [9]	185	89	5.9	44
Total	1405	93	3.0	59

Study data of disease-specific survival and recurrence after nephron-sparing surgery for localized renal cell carcinoma.

no recurrences at a median follow-up of 24 months. Of note, 28% of the resected lesions were benign. Kavoussi's group from Johns Hopkins published their experience in 48 patients with renal cell carcinoma [25]. The positive margin rate of 2.1% and local recurrence rate of 4.2% were comparable to series of open partial nephrectomies (Table 1). Cancer-specific survival was 100% with a mean follow-up of 37.7 months (range 22–84). In their most recent 50 patients, the positive margin rate was 0%. A landmark study from the Cleveland Clinic retrospectively compared 100 consecutive patients who underwent laparoscopic partial nephrectomy (LPN) from September 1999 with a similar cohort of 100 patients who underwent open partial nephrectomy from April 1998 [26]. All patients had a solitary renal tumor <7 cm. There was no difference in major postoperative complications. Open partial nephrectomy resulted in statistically significantly shorter warm ischemia times (17.5 vs 27.8 min), fewer intraoperative complications (0% vs 5%), and fewer urological postoperative complications (2% vs 11%). However, LPN offered a shorter hospital stay (2 vs 5 days), less postoperative pain (20 vs 253 morphine equivalents), and reduced convalescence (4 vs 6 weeks).

Because recurrence for open partial nephrectomy is highest during the first 3–5 years, the data for LPN still need to mature [34,35]. However, from the preliminary studies, oncologic control appears to be equivalent to open partial nephrectomy as well as to radical nephrectomy.

Indications

There are three indications for partial nephrectomy: absolute, relative, and elective [2,6]. Absolute indications include situations in which a radical nephrectomy would render a patient anephric with the need for immediate dialysis, for example in bilateral RCC or RCC in a solitary kidney. Relative indications include patients with a compromised contralateral kidney such that radical nephrectomy would increase their risk of renal insufficiency and possible renal failure, for example patients with nephrolithiasis, chronic pyelonephritis, renal artery stenosis, vesicoureteral reflux, or systemic diseases which affect the kidneys such as diabetes or hypertension. In addition, patients with hereditary RCC, such as von Hippel–Lindau disease, benefit from nephron-sparing surgery. Elective indications include patients with a single, localized unilateral renal tumor <4 cm and a normal contralateral kidney.

Indications for laparoscopic partial nephrectomy are the same as those for open partial nephrectomy. Contraindications include those that are universal for all laparoscopic surgery: uncorrected coagulopathy, untreated infection and bowel obstruction [36]. Precautions include prior abdominal or renal surgery, morbid obesity and ileus. In addition, endophytic tumors (<40% of tumor mass protruding above the surface of the kidney) and tumors close to the hilar vessels are more challenging and may better be addressed with standard open surgery dependent upon the surgeon's laparoscopic abilities. In contrast, exophytic lesions (i.e., >60% of the lesion protruding above the renal surface) and mesophytic lesions (i.e., >40% but <60% of the lesion protruding above the renal surface) are more easily approached laparoscopically.

Approach

Preoperative evaluation should include three-dimensional volume-rendered computerized tomography (CT) angiography to assess extent of disease, evaluate the renal vein/inferior vena cava, and determine the exact location and vascular supply of the tumor [37]. This single test combines data from angiography, venography, and excretory urography to outline the renal parenchyma and vasculature, obviating the need for invasive angiography.

Based on the CT findings, for small exophytic lesions (i.e., those for which hilar clamping is felt to not be necessary) a transperitoneal approach is employed if the lesion is anterior, anterolateral, lateral, or polar, while retroperitoneoscopy is reserved for posterior or posterolaterally located tumors (Fig. 1). If hilar clamping is planned, then a transperitoneal approach is used regardless of the tumor's location. Hand-assisted transperitoneal laparoscopy is favored by many urologists because it allows for tactile feedback and rapid hemostasis, and facilitates intracorporeal suturing. It has also been successfully applied to complex resections—multifocal or centrally located tumors (Fig. 1) [38]. Robotic-assisted LPN has just recently been reported [39]. Among 13 lesions the mean diameter was 3.5 cm (range 2.0–6.0), mean operative time was 3.6 h (range 2.2–4.4), and the mean blood loss was 170 ml (range 50–300). The mean warm ischemia was 22 min (range 15–29). The length of hospital stay averaged 4.3 days (range 2–7). There was one positive margin but a subsequent completion nephrectomy showed no evidence of residual tumor. One patient experienced

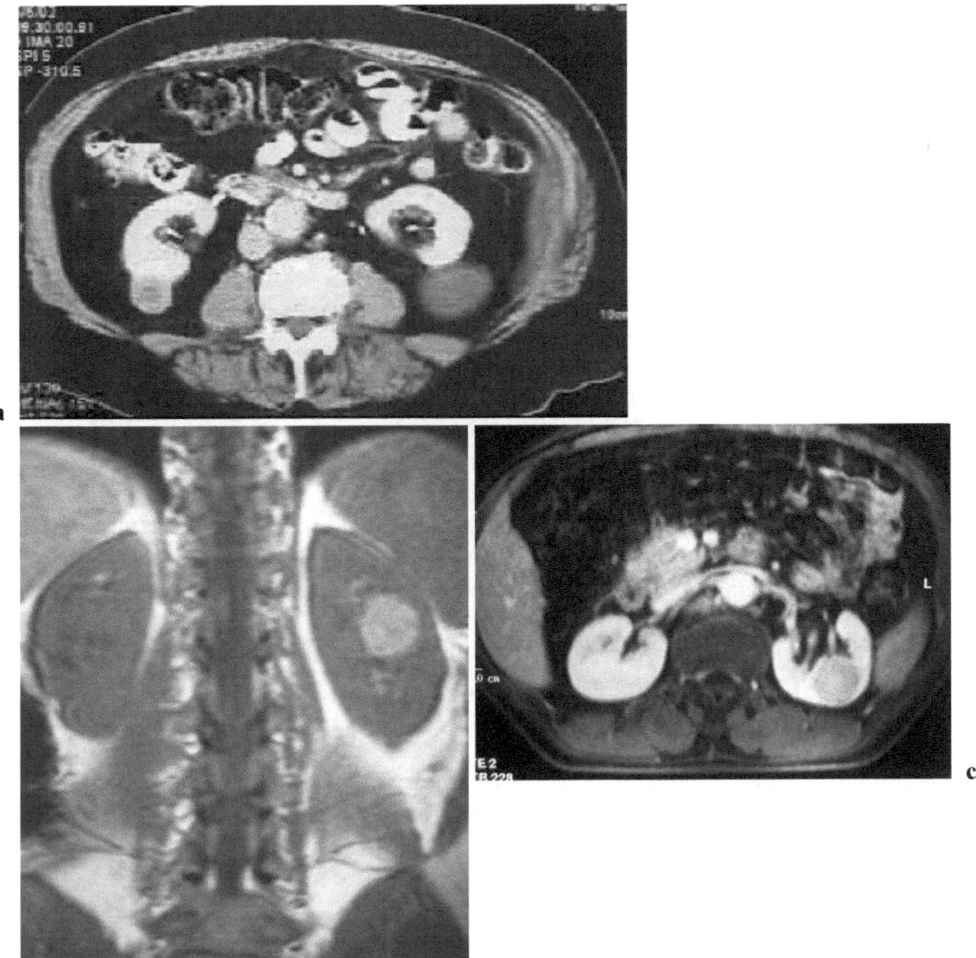

FIG. 1a–c. Tumors amenable to laparoscopic partial nephrectomy. **a** Computerized tomography scan demonstrating posterior tumors which can be addressed by a retroperitoneal approach. **b**,**c** Coronal and axial magnetic resonance images of an endophytic mass amenable to transperitoneal pure or hand-assisted laparoscopic partial nephrectomy

postoperative ileus. Although follow-up was short (2–11 months), there were no recurrences. The authors cautioned against a retroperitoneal approach if the robot was to be used.

Technique

Ureteral Catheters

In general, there is no need to place an external ureteral catheter or indwelling stent prior to partial nephrectomy even if entry into the collecting system is likely or planned. Indeed, in a landmark paper, Kavoussi and associates showed there was no benefit to ureteral catheter placement to identify caliceal entry [40]. In this retrospective study of 103 patients who underwent LPN for tumors <4.5 cm, 54 patients had intraoperative placement of a ureteral catheter to help identify collecting system entry via retrograde instillation of methylene blue, and 49 patients had no catheter. Operative time was significantly longer by 40 min in the ureteral catheter group. There was one instance of urinary fistula in each group requiring prolonged suction drainage. The authors concluded that laparoscopic magnification can identify collecting system entry and that a ureteral catheter may not decrease the instance of urinary fistula.

With cold incision of the parenchyma, the cut edge of the collecting system can usually be clearly seen and repaired. There is no benefit to "testing" the closure via an external stent; indeed, the closure may be blown out by such a maneuver. Similarly, placement of fibrin glue over the closed collecting system is not done in our practice, as this has a tendency to break down in three weeks and both of the leaks in our series were associated with the use of fibrin glue, despite achieving a watertight closure as demonstrated by retrograde injection of contrast via an external ureteral stent.

The transperitoneal and retroperitoneal approaches are identical to that described for a simple nephrectomy [23]. As such, the following comments assume that the organs surrounding the kidney have been properly mobilized and the surgeon is ready to treat the renal tumor.

Treating the Lesion Without Hilar Control

In general, this approach is limited to <3 cm exophytic or mesophytic lesions that do not extend more than 10 mm into the renal parenchyma, such that entry into the collecting system is unlikely. The exophytic renal lesion is identified both visually and with the aid of laparoscopic ultrasound. Gerota's fascia is sharply entered and the perinephric fat is cleared from around the tumor. With the aid of the ultrasound to mark the confines of the tumor, the renal capsule is scored with the hook electrocautery, floating ball electrode, or argon beam coagulator. Using the curved harmonic shears or the Ligasure device (Valleylab, Boulder, CO, USA) the circumferential incision is deepened until it lies below the meas-

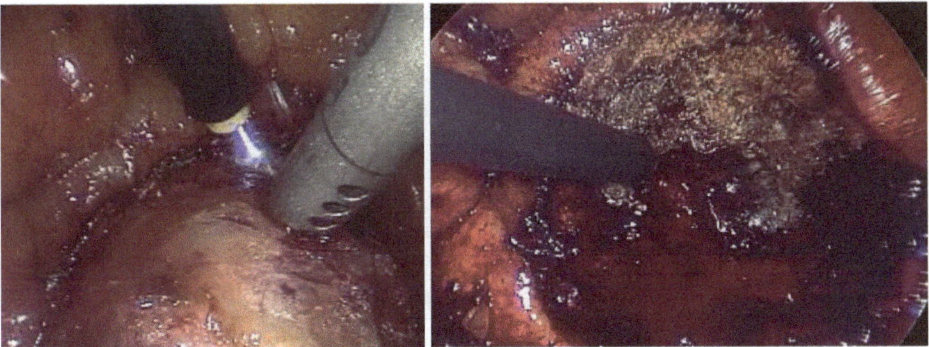

FIG. 2. Argon beam coagulator forming eschar at the base of a wedge resection

ured depth of the tumor by 3–5 mm. The tumor is then undermined and excised.

If the collecting system has not been entered, then the base of the tumor is treated with the argon beam coagulator followed by a layer of fibrin glue (Fig. 2). A patch of oxidized cellulose (e.g., Surgicel: Ethicon, Somerville, NJ, USA) is placed on top of the fibrin glue to further seal the cavity and then another layer of fibrin glue is placed on top of the oxidized cellulose, in a manner similar to that described by Wolf and colleagues [41].

If the collecting system has been entered, it is closed with a 6-inch running suture of 2-0 Vicryl on an SH needle; a Lapra-Ty clip (Ethicon) is placed on the free end of the suture before it is introduced into the abdominal cavity. After several throws, the collecting system should be closed. A Lapra-Ty clip is advanced along the taut end of the running suture until it lies flush with the renal parenchyma, and is then fixed in place. As such, no intracorporeal knot tying is needed. At this point, a layer of hemostatic gelatin matrix (e.g., Floseal: Baxter Healthcare, Irvine, CA, USA) is applied to the tumor bed. The pneumoperitoneum is lowered to 5 mmHg to check for hemostasis.

Hilar Control

On either side, the renal artery and renal vein can be separately dissected, as one would do for a radical nephrectomy, and occluded with laparoscopic bulldog clamps. Alternatively, if one is planning to clamp both the artery and vein en bloc with a Satinsky clamp, the area of the hilum need only be roughed out by dissecting the anterior surface of the vein, and the area posterior to the vessels. The entire hilar mass of tissue can then be secured with the Satinsky clamp. The clamp can be introduced via a separate 5 mm incision in the pararectus line, inferior to the umbilicus so as to provide a smooth and direct path to the renal hilum.

It is our practice to clamp only the artery as it has been suggested that complete hilar occlusion is more damaging to the kidney, although this has not been adequately demonstrated [6,42]. The surgeon should consider placing two bulldogs on the renal artery in order to achieve complete occlusion; one is often not sufficient (J. Landman, personal communication, 2005). The lesion is excised using a 5-mm Ligasure device, harmonic shears or cold scissors, aiming for a 5-mm margin. The argon beam coagulator is used to form a thin layer of eschar on the cut surface of the renal parenchyma. For very small, exophytic lesions, this along with a fibrin glue/Surgicel/fibrin glue sandwich may suffice for hemostasis. For larger defects, with entry into the collecting system, a more formal closure is needed. Closure of the collecting system is as previously described using a running suture of 0-Vicyrl on an SH needle; Lapra-Ty clips are used to secure the suture at either end.

Next, absorbable bolster(s) of oxidized regenerated cellulose, tied at either end with a 0-Chromic tie, are used (e.g., Surgicel Nu-Knit wrapped around Surgicel absorbable hemostat [Ethicon]). We use a modification of Shalhav's technique to close the renal parenchyma over the bolster(s) without the need for intracorporeal knot tying [30]. A 10-inch length of 0-Vicryl suture on a CT-1 needle is anchored with a Lapra-Ty clip. Suturing is easiest with the needle driver entering the abdomen parallel to the renal defect; as such the camera and instrument ports are shifted accordingly. The kidney is fixed in position with a 5-mm PEER retractor (Jarit Surgical Instruments, Hawthorne, NY, USA) attached to an Endoholder device (Codman, Raynham, MA, USA). A simple suture is placed to bridge the most distal portion of the wound first. Starting 5–10 mm below the cut surface of the kidney, the needle is driven through the renal capsule and into the defect and passed into and over the bolster. By taking a small bite of the bolster, it remains in place on the kidney surface (as per A. Belldegrun, personal communication, 2004). The needle is then passed through the opposite side of the defect, out through the renal capsule. With the suture held taut and perpendicular to the kidney, a Lapra-Ty clip is placed flush against the renal capsule to secure the stitch in place. Immediately, a second Lapra-Ty clip is placed 1 cm distal to the first and the suture is cut between the two clips (Fig. 3). Thus, a second interrupted suture can be placed without delay. Usually, 3–4 separate sutures can be obtained using the one 10-inch length of suture, thereby eliminating time consuming entry and removal of multiple sutures and needles. The process is completed until the defect is closed. At this point, a generous layer of FloSeal is placed over the area of closure. The bulldog clamp(s) or Satinsky clamp is removed and the pneumoperitoneum is reduced to 5 mmHg to help identify small bleeders.

Hand-Assisted

The hand-assist port can be placed in the midline, and the port placement changed accordingly [32]. Any of the hand assist devices may be used. This approach simplifies suturing as well as hemostasis and specimen retrieval.

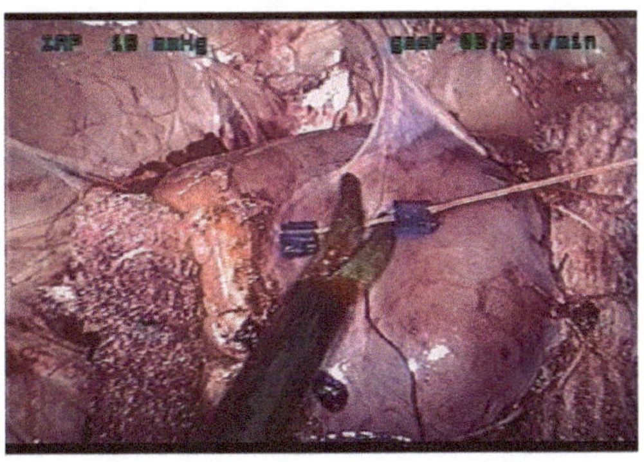

FIG. 3. Lapra-Ty assisted closure of the renal parenchyma in a porcine kidney

Specimen Retrieval

As soon as hemostasis is obtained, a plastic entrapment sack is placed and the lesion entrapped. One port site is extended to 2cm to allow removal of the specimen. A blunt port with an inflatable balloon retention mechanism can then be placed to re-establish the pneumoperitoneum. The specimen is sent for frozen section. If the margins are not clear, then the fibrin glue/Surgicel patch is removed and additional tissue is taken, using the harmonic shears to deliver another 2mm "rind" deep to the original resection bed. Fortunately, in our experience as well as others, the need to do this is rare [25,43].

Surgical Margin

The minimum clear margin necessary after resection of renal cancers now appears to be 2.5–5mm, rather than the traditional 10mm. In 63 patients who underwent partial nephrectomy with 10-mm margins, Zucchi et al. reported a 6% incidence of satellite lesions with a mean distance of 5.3mm from the primary lesion [44]. In contrast, Li et al. sectioned 82 kidneys with small renal cell carcinomas at 3-mm intervals [45]. They noted that the chance of tumor recurrence when the margin is at least 2.5mm is only 1.2%. Likewise, Sutherland et al. analyzed recurrence rates and surgical margin size after partial nephrectomy for $T_{1-2}N_0M_0$ RCC among 41 patients with negative margins [46]. Mean and median surgical margin was 2.5 and 2.0mm, respectively. After a mean follow-up of 4 years there were no local recurrences. However, small low-grade renal cell cancers may take far more than 4 years to grow to a radiographically detectable size given the reported average growth rate for renal cell carcinoma of 1–4mm per year [47,48]. Even more extreme than a 2.5-mm margin is no margin at all; some studies have demonstrated no increased risk of local recurrence with open enucleation of low-stage tumors [11,46]. This practice is generally to be eschewed, except in the setting of hereditary RCC. In sum, minimal margins of 2.5–5 mm of normal renal parenchyma appear adequate to prevent local tumor recurrence and enable maximal nephron sparing in the vast majority of cases.

Warm and Cold Ischemia: Concerns and Limits

The length of acceptable warm ischemia time (WIT) and the need for renal cooling are both based largely on historical evidence [49,50]. Ward's seminal canine studies demonstrated tolerance to warm ischemia up to 30 min with 60%–70% acute diminution of renal function, but complete recovery within one week. Warm ischemia times of >60 min resulted in delayed return of function of several weeks, and >120 min resulted in significant, irreversible renal damage. Acute tubular necrosis is the second most common complication after nephron sparing surgery, occurring in a mean of 6.3% of patients [51].

Recently, Guillonneau et al. compared the mean difference between pre- and one month postoperative serum creatinine after LPN with and without vessel clamping in 28 unmatched patients [28]. With an average clamp time of only 27.3 ± 7 min (range 15–47 min) they found a change in serum creatinine at one month of 0.2 mg/dl in the clamped group vs 0.09 mg/dl in the unclamped group ($P = 0.052$), despite similar size renal lesions in both groups (2.5 vs 2.0 cm). Operative time and estimated blood loss were statistically significantly less in the clamped group (121.5 min and 270 ml vs 179.1 min and 708 ml). Argon bean coagulation, fibrin glue, FloSeal, and other hemostatic agents were not used. The authors concluded that the main advantage of renal vascular clamping was the ability to visualize the renal parenchyma, thus facilitating accurate tumor excision by clear identification of the mass and surgical margins.

In the Cleveland Clinic series comparing 100 laparoscopic and 100 open nephron-sparing procedures, vascular clamping was performed in 97% of cases in the laparoscopic group, with an average warm ischemia time of 27.8 min [26]. Although the reported change in creatinine was minimal (0.10 mg/dl), in a subset of patients with a solitary kidney ($n = 7$), the change in creatinine within 1 month of surgery was 0.50 mg/dl.

While most groups report warm ischemia times of just under 30 min, this historical cutoff has recently been challenged. In a series from Johns Hopkins, 118 patients who underwent LPN for a single, unilateral renal tumor with a normal contralateral kidney were retrospectively stratified into three groups based on the amount of warm ischemia time: no ischemia (42), <30 min (48) and >30 min (28) [31]. At six months, there was no statistically significant difference in the mean change in creatinine (0.05, 0.06, 0.08) and all patients who underwent imaging via CT or magnetic resonance imaging (MRI) ($n = 114$) demonstrated prompt, symmetric excretion during the nephrogenic phase. Although the decision to obtain vascular control was subjective, based on patient and tumor characteristics in this retrospective study, these results do suggest that warm ischemia times of greater than 30 min—up to 55 min in this series—can be tolerated with no adverse effects on renal function. Other retrospective studies have shown similar tolerance to warm ischemia greater than 30 min [52,53].

Two groups have taken the question of tolerance to warm ischemia to the laboratory using a solitary kidney pig model. Baldwin et al. performed laparoscopic nephrectomy on 16 pigs [54]. Two weeks later, the contralateral renal hilum was clamped for 0, 30, 60, or 90 min. Serum creatinine was monitored for 4 weeks. They found that the pigs who underwent WIT of 60 and 90 min experienced transient increases in creatinine which resolved by one week. Laven et al. performed laparoscopic nephrectomy on 32 pigs [55]. Twelve days later, they were divided into four subgroups of 0, 30, 60, and 90 min of WIT. While pigs in the 60-min and 90-min groups experienced a transient decrease in renal function at 72 h, by day 15 there were no differences among any of the groups. Together, these studies suggest that warm ischemia times of up to 90 min produce no permanent renal impairment.

Cold Ischemia/Renal Cooling

For complex resections that are estimated to require more than 30 min or for already compromised renal units, some authors recommend duplicating the open practice of renal hypothermia [51]. This may extend the ischemic time to as long as 3 h without irreversible renal damage [49]. Ward suggested that optimal renal protection could be achieved at temperatures below 15°C [50]. There are three primary access points to achieve renal hypothermia: renal capsule, renal hilum, and collecting system. Gill et al. reported clamping the renal hilum and then using ice slush in a plastic entrapment sack to achieve renal hypothermia with a nadir temperature range of 5°–19°C [56,57]. The opening of the bag is brought out through a port site to facilitate filling with ice slush for 10 min, after which time the bag is removed and tumor resection begins. In 12 patients they noted a mean warm ischemia time of 4 min and mean total ischemia time of 43.5 min. All kidneys functioned on postoperative renal scan. Based on this technique, others have designed machines to produce finely chopped ice which is pumped through a laparoscopic port [58] or have employed continuous irrigation of perirenal gauze sponges with cold saline [38]; however, neither approach has been used clinically as of yet.

A second method of cooling is achieved via a vascular approach. During open partial nephrectomy, Munver et al. cannulated the renal artery and vein of nine patients using a 14-gauge catheter and infused lactated Ringer's solution cooled to 4°C [59]. They were able to achieve rapid renal cooling (within 2 min), although absolute temperatures were not reported. Subsequently, in 15 patients undergoing LPN, Janetschek et al. had an angiocatheter placed in the renal artery through a femoral puncture preoperatively [60]. At the time of hilar occlusion, they perfused the kidney with iced lactated Ringer's solution and achieved renal hypothermia of 25°C. Mean ischemia time was 40 min. Follow-up studies in 11 patients showed no significant decrease in renal function. This is a rather tedious and potentially problematic method, and has not become popular in the United States.

Finally, renal parenchymal cooling via cold saline perfusion of the collecting system was originally reported by Jones and Politano in 1963 [61]. This approach has been adapted in animal models via retrograde placement of a dual-lumen catheter [62] or a ureteral access sheath [63]. In both studies, this method was unable to cool the renal parenchyma below 26°C and 21°C, respectively. However, using a porcine model Landman and associates noted histologic preservation of renal parenchyma after 30 min of cold ischemia in contradistinction to a warm ischemia control group which manifested significant cortical and medullary inflammation with periarteriolar hemorrhage. Of note, these groups did report colder medullary cooling temperatures, compared to cortical temperatures, which is not surprising given the inside-out method of cooling that is used with this approach. However, with all of these animal studies, it is sobering to realize that warm ischemia out to 90 min is well tolerated in pigs and thus calls into question whether cold ischemia is indeed of any benefit in this animal model.

Hemostasis

There has been tremendous progress in the area of hemostasis with regard to partial nephrectomy. Three groups of agents exist to help in this regard: hemostatic preparations, sealants, and glues. The first is exemplified by substances such as oxidized regenerated cellulose, absorbable gelatin, or microfibrillar collagen. More recently thrombin impregnated collagen beads (e.g., FloSeal) have been used to stop bleeding even in the presence of a "wet" environment (i.e., some ongoing oozing). However, they cannot seal an open collecting system. In contrast, fibrin glue (e.g., Tisseel: Baxter) is actually not a glue, but a hemostatic sealant. It consists of human fibrinogen and thrombin plus bovine aprotinin, a fibrinolysis inhibitor, which create an adherent clot when mixed. Of note, this works well only in a "dry" environment so it does not get diluted as it is applied. The third option is a true tissue glue. Examples of this include cyanoacrylate, polyethylene glycol-based hydrogel, and albumin/glutaraldehyde (BioGlue: CryoLife, Kennesaw, GA, USA). These materials only work under conditions of hemostasis with a totally dry surface. They have no formal hemostatic properties but instead adhere to the tissue. Once dry, vessels are sealed and do not bleed. To date, LPN work with tissue glues has been limited to animal studies [64].

Other Energy Sources

Multiple authors have sought in vain a way to "carve" the kidney in a bloodless fashion without hilar control. To date, none have succeeded. Clayman and colleagues developed a hollow wire-cutting snare that could perform a "bloodless" polar nephrectomy in pigs [65]. Unfortunately, this has never come to clinical trials due to industry disinterest. Cadeddu and colleagues have used the holmium laser successfully to cut into the porcine kidney [66]; however, again the pig turned out to be a kinder model than the human and when taken to human trials it did not perform well. Similarly, floating-ball monopolar wet electrosurgery (TissueLink Medical, Dover, NH, USA) has come onto the scene. Initial series noted no vascular clamping; however, as authors have gained more experience with this device and approached larger or more endophytic lesions, the recommendation to clamp the vessels has been voiced [67–70]. Finally, in Japan, Terai and colleagues used a microwave probe to coagulate the peritumor area prior to excision [71]. While this worked in 18 patients the technique resulted in collecting system strictures in one patient, which resulted in eventual renal loss.

Postoperative Care

In the literature, a drain is placed at the end of partial nephrectomy, whether open or laparoscopic. We use a 5-mm round drain placed in the lateral most port. A Foley catheter is placed. No indwelling stent is placed in any case regardless of entry into the collecting system. In this regard, we have adopted Shalhav's postoperative routine regarding drain management [30]. Specifically, as soon as the drainage is less than 50cc for an 8-h shift, the Foley catheter is removed. If the drainage over two consecutive 8-h shifts remains at less than 50cc per shift, then the drain is removed and the patient can be discharged.

Complications

The main complications of laparoscopic partial nephrectomy are bleeding and urinary leak (Table 2). Kim et al. compared 114 consecutive patients undergoing either LPN (35) or laparoscopic radical nephrectomy (79) and found no statistically significant difference in the surgical complication rate (19.7% vs 17.5%) while overall complications were 12.7% vs 34.3% [29]. The Cleveland Clinic study comparing 100 LPN with 100 open partial nephrectomies found no statistically significant difference in the overall number of complications, 19% vs 13% [26]. However, LPN had more major intraoperative incidents (5% vs 0%), and more renal or urinary tract injury (11% vs 2%, urinary fistula 3% vs 1%). In a recent review of 200 LPNs at the Cleveland Clinic, there was a 33% overall complication rate, including a hemorrhage rate of 9.5% [33]. Overall, 4.5% had urine leakage, which was managed conservatively in all cases either by stent placement with or without percutaneous drainage of the urinoma, or observation. In addition, 15% of the complications were nonurological, including pulmonary (5%) and cardiovascular (4.5%).

TABLE 2. Selected series of laparoscopic partial nephrectomy with ≥25 patients since 2000

First author [Ref.]	No. of patients	Mean tumor size (cm)	Hilar control?	Collecting system repair (%)	Hemostasis technique	Mean blood loss (ml)	Mean operative time (h)	Mean hospital stay (days)
Janetschek [27]	25	1.9	No	0	Bipolar, argon beam, glue	287	2.7	5.8
Rassweiler [24]	53	2.3	—	—	Harmonic, bipolar, argon beam, Nd:YAG	725	3.2	5.4
Gill [26]	100	2.8	Yes (91)	64	Suture over bolsters	125	3.0	2.0
Guillonneau [28]	28	1.9	No (12)	0	Bipolar, harmonic	708	3.0	4.7
		2.5	Yes (16)	11	Suture over bolsters	270	2.0	4.7
Kim [29]	79	2.5	Yes (52)	—	Suture over bolsters	391	3.0	2.8
Orvieto [30]	32	2.2	Yes (29)	66	Argon beam, fibrin glue, suture over bolster	223	3.7	2.7
Bhayani [31]	42	2.4	No	—	—	390	3.2	2.9
	76	2.6	Yes	—	—	354	2.7	2.7
Strup [32]	32	2.6	Sometimes	—	Argon beam, fibrin glue patch, sutures	400	3.6	3.8
Allaf [25]	48	2.4	Yes	—	Suture over bolsters	—	—	—
Ramani [33]	200	2.9	Yes	71	Suture over bolsters, FloSeal	247	3.3	—
Total	715	2.4	—	—	—	375	3.0	3.8

The table details results of recently published series of laparoscopic partial nephrectomy.

The Future (Minimally Invasive Ablation)

Laparoscopy is dying! The future of tissue ablation lies in percutaneous image-guided (i.e., CT, MRI, and/or ultrasound) ablation using either cryotherapy or radiofrequency (RF) probes. With cryotherapy, both laparoscopic and percutaneous, there have been no occurrences of metastatic disease or cancer deaths in hundreds of patients with follow-up out to 4 years. Radiofrequency has had a more checkered record due to incomplete treatment of lesions in two series and to collecting system injury in a few cases, and to the variation in power of the devices used [72,73]. However, the 200-W RF needles appear to be far more effective than their less powerful predecessors. Nonetheless, this is where the future lies, in our opinion. But even percutaneous ablation itself may begin to wane if noninvasive high-intensity focused ultrasound (HIFU) comes to fruition. While early results from Alken's group in Germany were promising, there were no reports of complete tumor death [74]. Likewise, Marberger et al. applied HIFU to 14 patients; at the time of tumor harvest, all 14 had residual tumor [75]! Despite these dismal results, one has to believe that advances in technology will eventually provide us with an effective extracorporeal modality for tissue ablation.

Conclusion

Laparoscopic partial nephrectomy is a technically challenging procedure that is still in its infancy. While further refinements in hemostatic devices and sealants will facilitate more widespread adoption of LPN, the future may ultimately lie with less invasive techniques such as percutaneous needle ablation and noninvasive tissue ablation. Surgical cure without a surgical incursion remains the goal; we are not there yet, but the end is in sight.

References

1. Hock LM, Lynch J, Balaji KC (2002) Increasing incidence of all stages of kidney cancer in the last two decades in the United States: an analysis of surveillance, epidemiology and end results program data. J Urol 167:57–60
2. Novick AC (2004) Laparoscopic and partial nephrectomy. Clin Cancer Res 10:6322s–6327s
3. Clayman RV, Kavoussi LR, Soper NJ, Dierks SM, Meretyk S, Darcy MD, Long SR, Roemer FD, Pingleton ED, Thompson PG (1991) Laparoscopic nephrectomy. N Engl J Med 324:1370–1371
4. Clayman RV, Kavoussi LR, Soper NJ, Dierks SM, Meretyk S, Darcy MD, Roemer FD, Pingleton ED, Thompson PG, Long SR (1991) Laparoscopic nephrectomy: initial case report. J Urol 146:278–282
5. Zisman A, Pantuck AJ, Belldegrun AS, Schulam PG (2001) Laparoscopic radical nephrectomy. Semin Urol Oncol 19:114–122

6. Novick AC (2002) Surgery of the kidney. In: Walsh PC, Retik AB, Vaughn ED, Wein AJ (eds) Campbell's urology, 8th edn. Saunders, Philadelphia, pp 3570–3643
7. Lee CT, Katz J, Shi W, Thaler HT, Reuter VE, Russo P (2000) Surgical management of renal tumors 4 cm. or less in a contemporary cohort. J Urol 163:730–736
8. Hafez KS, Novick AC, Butler BP (1998) Management of small solitary unilateral renal cell carcinomas: impact of central versus peripheral tumor location. J Urol 159:1156–1160
9. Lerner SE, Hawkins CA, Blute ML, Grabner A, Wollan PC, Eickholt JT, Zincke H (2002) Disease outcome in patients with low stage renal cell carcinoma treated with nephron sparing or radical surgery. J Urol 167:884–889
10. McKiernan J, Simmons R, Katz J, Russo P (2002) Natural history of chronic renal insufficiency after partial and radical nephrectomy. Urology 59:816–820
11. Lau WK, Blute ML, Weaver AL, Torres VE, Zincke H (2000) Matched comparison of radical nephrectomy vs nephron-sparing surgery in patients with unilateral renal cell carcinoma and a normal contralateral kidney. Mayo Clin Proc 75:1236–1242
12. Moll V, Becht E, Zigler M (1993) Kidney preserving surgery in renal cell tumors: indications, techniques and results in 152 patients. J Urol 150:319–323
13. Steinbach F, Stockle M, Hohenfellner R (1995) Clinical experience with nephron-sparing surgery in the presence of a normal contralateral kidney. Semin Urol Oncol 13:288–291
14. D'Armiento M, Damiano R, Felepa B, Perdona S, Oriani G, De Sio M (1997) Elective conservative surgery for renal carcinoma versus radical nephrectomy: a prospective study. Br J Urol 79:15–19
15. Hafez KS, Fergany AF, Novick AC (1999) Nephron sparing surgery for localized renal cell carcinoma: impact of tumor size on patient survival, tumor recurrence and TNM staging. J Urol 162:1930–1933
16. Barbalias GA, Liatsikos EN, Tsintayis A, Nikiforidis G (1999) Adenocarcinoma of the kidney: nephron-sparing surgical approach vs radical nephrectomy. J Surg Oncol 72:156–161
17. Belldegrun A, Tsui KH, deKernion JB, Smith RB (1997) Efficacy of nephron-sparing surgery for renal cell carcinoma: analysis based on the new 1997 Tumor-Node-Metastasis Staging System. J Clin Oncol 17:2868–2875
18. Herr HW (1999) Partial nephrectomy for unilateral renal carcinoma and a normal contralateral kidney: 10-year followup. J Urol 161:33–34
19. Fergany AF, Hafez KS, Novick AC (2000) Long-term results of nephron-sparing surgery for localized renal cell carcinoma: 10 year follow-up. J Urol 163:442–445
20. Winfield HN, Donovan JF, Godet AS, Clayman RV (1993) Laparoscopic partial nephrectomy: initial case report for benign disease. J Endourol 7:521–526
21. McDougall EM, Clayman RV, Chandhoke PS, Kerbl K, Stone AM, Wick MR, Hicks M, Figenshau RS (1993) Laparoscopic partial nephrectomy in the pig model. J Urol 149:1633–1636
22. McDougall EM, Clayman RV, Anderson K (1993) Laparoscopic wedge resection of a renal tumor: initial experience. J Laparoendosc Surg 3:577–581
23. Gill IS, Delworth MG, Munch LC (1994) Laparoscopic retroperitoneal partial nephrectomy. J Urol 152:1539–1542
24. Rassweiler JJ, Abbou C, Janetschek G, Jeschke K (2000) Laparoscopic partial nephrectomy. The European experience. Urol Clin North Am 27:721–736

25. Allaf ME, Bhayani SB, Rogers C, Varkarakis I, Link RE, Inagaki T, Jarrett TW, Kavoussi LR (2004) Laparoscopic partial nephrectomy: evaluation of long-term oncological outcome. J Urol 172:871–873
26. Gill IS, Matin SF, Desai MM, Kaouk JH, Steinberg A, Mascha E, Thornton J, Sherief MH, Strzempkowski B, Novick AC (2003) Comparative analysis of laparoscopic versus open partial nephrectomy for renal tumors in 200 patients. J Urol 170:64–68
27. Janetschek G, Jeschke K, Peschel R, Strohmeyer D, Henning K, Bartsch G (2000) Laparoscopic surgery for stage T1 renal cell carcinoma: radical nephrectomy and wedge resection. Eur Urol 38:131–138
28. Guillonneau B, Bermudez H, Gholami S, Fettouh HE, Gupta R, Rosa JA, Baumert H, Cathelineau X, Fromont G, Vallancien G (2003) Laparoscopic partial nephrectomy for renal tumor: single center experience comparing clamping and no clamping techniques of the renal vasculature. J Urol 169:483–486
29. Kim FJ, Rha KH, Hernandez F, Jarrett TW, Pinto PA, Kavoussi LR (2003) Laparoscopic radical versus partial nephrectomy: assessment of complications. J Urol 170:408–411
30. Orvieto MA, Chein GW, Laven B Rapp DE, Sokoloff MH, Shalhav AL (2004) Eliminating knot tying during warm ischemia time for laparoscopic partial nephrectomy. J Urol 172:2292–2295
31. Bhayani SB, Rha KH, Pinto PA, Ong AM, Allaf ME, Trock BJ, Jarrett TW, Kavoussi LR (2004) Laparoscopic partial nephrectomy: effect of warm ischemia on serum creatinine. J Urol 172:1264–1266
32. Strup SE, Hubosky S (2004) Hand-assisted laparoscopic partial nephrectomy. J Endourol 18:345–349
33. Ramani AP, Desai MM, Steinberg AP Ng CS, Abreu SC, Kaouk JH, Finelli A, Novick AC, Gill IS (2005) Complications of laparoscopic partial nephrectomy in 200 cases. J Urol 173:42–47
34. Hafez KS, Novick AC, Campbell SC (1997) Patterns of tumor recurrence and guidelines for followup after nephron-sparing surgery for sporadic renal cell carcinoma. J Urol 157:2067–2070
35. Montie JE (1994) Follow-up after partial or total nephrectomy for renal cell carcinoma. Urol Clin North Am 21:589–592
36. Capeluto CC, Kavoussi LR (1993) Complications of laparoscopic surgery. Urology 42:2–12
37. Coll DM, Uzzo RG, Herts BR, Davros WJ, Wirth SL, Novick AC (1999) 3-dimensional volume rendered computerized tomography for preoperative evaluation and intraoperative treatment of patients undergoing nephron sparing surgery. J Urol 161:1097–1102
38. Herrell SD (2004) Laparoscopic partial nephrectomy techniques: developments and translation. J Urol 172:2553–2556
39. Gettman MT, Blute ML, Chow GK, Neururer R, Bartsch G, Peschel R (2004) Robotic-assisted laparoscopic partial nephrectomy: technique and initial clinical experience with DaVinci robotic system. Urology 64:914–918
40. Bove P, Bhayani SB, Rha KH, Allaf ME, Jarrett TW, Kavoussi LR (2004) Necessity of ureteral catheter during laparoscopic partial nephrectomy. J Urol 172:458–460
41. Wolf JS Jr, Seifman BD, Montie JE (2000) Nephron sparing surgery for suspected malignancy: open surgery compared to laparoscopy with selective use of hand assistance. J Urol 163:1659–1664

42. Nadelhaft P, Nimmermann A, Bishop MC (1981) Arterial and pedicle occlusion in the hypothermic pig kidney. Urol Res 9:169–173
43. Kubinski DJ, Clark PE, Assimos DG, Hall MC (2004) Utility of frozen section analysis of resection margins during partial nephrectomy. Urology 64:31–34
44. Zucchi A, Mearini L, Mearini E Costantini E, Vivacqua C, Porena M (2003) Renal cell carcinoma: histological findings on surgical margins after nephron-sparing surgery. J Urol 169:905–908
45. Li QL, Guan HW, Zhang LZ, Zhang LZ, Wang FP, Liu YJ (2003) Optimal margin in nephron-sparing surgery for renal cell carcinoma 4 cm or less in diameter. Eur Urol 44:448–451
46. Sutherland SE, Resnick MI, Maclennan GT, Goldman HB (2002) Does the size of the surgical margin in partial nephrectomy for renal cell cancer really matter? J Urol 167:61–64
47. Volpe A, Panzarella T, Rendon RA, Haider MA, Kondylis FI, Jewett MA (2004) The natural history of incidentally detected small renal masses. Cancer 100:738–745
48. Bosniak MA, Birnbaum BA, Krinsky GA, Waisman J (1995) Small renal parenchymal neoplasms: further observations on growth. Radiology 197:589–597
49. Novick AC (1983) Renal hypothermia: in vivo and ex vivo. Urol Clin North Am 10:637–644
50. Ward JP (1975) Determination of the optimum temperature for regional hypothermia during temporary renal ischemia. Br J Urol 47:17–24
51. Uzzo RG, Novick AC (2001) Nephron sparing surgery for renal tumors: indications, techniques and outcomes. J Urol 166:6–18
52. Wahlberg E, Dimuzio PJ, Stoney RJ (2002) Aortic clamping during elective operations for infrarenal disease: the influence of clamping time on renal function. J Vasc Surg 36:13–18
53. Nicholson ML, Metcalfe MS, White SA, Waller JR, Doughman TM, Horsburgh T, Feehally J, Carr SJ, Veitch PS (2000) A comparison of the results of renal transplantation from non-heart-beating, conventional cadaveric, and living donors. Kidney Int 58:2585–2591
54. Baldwin DD, Maynes LJ, Berger KA, Desai PJ, Zuppan CW, Zimmerman GJ, Winkielman AM, Sterling TH, Tsai CK, Ruckle HC (2004) Laparoscopic warm renal ischemia in the solitary porcine kidney model. Urology 63:592–597
55. Laven BA, Orvieto MA, Chuang MS, Ritch CR, Murray P, Harland RC, Inman SR, Brendler CB, Shalhav AL (2004) Renal tolerance to prolonged warm ischemia time in a laparoscopic versus open surgery porcine model. J Urol 172:2471–2474
56. Gill IS, Desai MM, Kaouk JH, Meraney AM, Murphy DP, Sung GT, Novick AC (2002) Laparoscopic partial nephrectomy for renal tumor: duplicating open surgical techniques. J Urol 167:469–470
57. Gill IS, Abreu SC, Desai MM, Steinberg AP, Ramani AP, Ng C, Banks K, Novick AC, Kaouk JH (2003) Laparoscopic ice slush renal hypothermia for partial nephrectomy: the initial experience. J Urol 170:52–56
58. Ames CD, Venkatesh R, Weld KJ, Perrone M, Landman J (2004) Laparoscopic renal parenchymal hypothermia with a novel ice-slush deployment mechanism. J Endourol 18:A7
59. Munver R, Threatt CB, Robertson CN (2003) Intra-arterial renal hypothermia for nephron-sparing surgery: initial experience and long-term follow-up. J Urol 169:4

60. Janetschek G, Al-Zahrani H, Vrabec G, Al-Zahrani H, Leeb K, Gschwendtner M (2003) Laparoscopic partial nephrectomy in cold ischemia: renal artery perfusion. J Urol 171:68–71
61. Jones WR, Politano V (1963) The effects of renal artery occlusion on renal function under normothermic and regional hypothermia. J Urol 89:535–541
62. Crain DS, Spencer CR, Favata MA, Amling CL (2004) Transureteral saline perfusion to obtain renal hypothermia: potential application in laparoscopic partial nephrectomy. J Soc Laparosc Surg 8:217–222
63. Landman J, Rehman J, Sundaram CP, Bhayani S, Monga M, Pattaras JG, Gokden N, Humphrey PA, Clayman RV (2002) Renal hypothermia achieved by retrograde intracavitary saline perfusion. J Endourol 16:445–449
64. Park EL, Ulreich JB, Scott KM, Ullrich NP, Linehan JA, French MH, Ho WY, White MJ, Talley JR, Fellah AM, Ramakumar S (2004) Evaluation of polyethylene glycol based hydrogel for tissue sealing after laparoscopic partial nephrectomy in a porcine model. J Urol 172:2446–2450
65. Collyer WC, Landman J, Olweny EO, Andreoni C, Kibel A, Andriole GL, Bostwick DG, Sundaram CP, Clayman RV (2002) Laparoscopic partial nephrectomy with a novel electrosurgical snare in a porcine model. J Endourol 16:673–679
66. Lotan Y, Gettman MT, Lindberg G, Napper CA, Hoopman J, Pearle MS, Cadeddu JA (2004) Laparoscopic partial nephrectomy using holmium laser in a porcine model. J Soc Laparosc Surg 8:51–55
67. Sundaram CP, Rehman J, Venkatesh R, Lee D, Rageb MM, Kibel A, Landman J (2003) Hemostatic laparoscopic partial nephrectomy assisted by a water-cooled, high-density, monopolar device without renal vascular control. Urology 61:906–909
68. Urena R, Mendez F, Woods M, Thomas R, Davis R (2004) Laparoscopic partial nephrectomy of solid renal masses without hilar clamping using a monopolar radio frequency device. J Urol 171:1054–1056
69. Stern JA, Simon SD, Ferrigni RG, Andrews PE (2004) TissueLink device for laparoscopic nephron-sparing surgery. J Endourol 18:455–456
70. Tan YH, Young MD, L'Esperance JO, Preminger GM, Albala DM (2004) Hand-assisted laparoscopic partial nephrectomy without hilar vascular clamping using a saline-cooled, high-density monopolar radiofrequency device. J Endourol 18:883–887
71. Terai A, Ito N, Yoshimura K, Ichioka K, Kamoto T, Arai Y, Ogawa O (2004) Laparoscopic partial nephrectomy using microwave tissue coagulator for small renal tumors: usefulness and complications. Eur Urol 45:744–748
72. Michaels MJ, Rhee HK, Mourtzinos AP, Summerhayes IC, Silverman ML, Libertino JA (2002) Incomplete renal tumor destruction using radio frequency interstitial ablation. J Urol 168:2046–2049
73. Rendon RA, Kachura JR, Sweet JM (2002) The uncertainty of radiofrequency treatment of renal cell carcinoma: findings at intermediate and delayed nephrectomy. J Urol 167:1587–1592
74. Kohrmann KU, Michel MS, Gaa J, Marlinghaus E, Alken P (2002) High intensity focused ultrasound as noninvasive therapy for multilocal renal cell carcinoma: case study and review of the literature. J Urol 167:2397–2403
75. Marberger M, Schatzl G, Cranston D, Kennedy JE (2005) Extracorporeal ablation of renal tumours with high-intensity focused ultrasound. BJU Int 95:52–55

Part 2
Upper Urinary Tract Tumor

Percutaneous Approach to Transitional Cell Carcinoma of the Upper Urinary Tract

BENG JIT TAN[1], MICHAEL C. OST[1], ROBERT MARCOVICH[2], BENJAMIN R. LEE[1], and ARTHUR D. SMITH[1]

Summary. The preliminary rationale for endoscopic management of upper tract transitional cell carcinoma (UTTCC) was to preserve renal parenchyma and to decrease the morbidity of therapy. In this regard, endoscopic management was introduced to treat patients with UTTCC in an anatomic or functional solitary kidney, patients with bilateral disease, and patients who were not candidates for open surgery due to underlying comorbidity. Today, endoscopic management remains the standard of care for such patients, as long as they have noninvasive disease. A percutaneous approach, in particular, has proven to be an effective minimally invasive treatment for large (>1.5 cm), low-grade UTTCC limited to the calices, renal pelvis, and proximal ureter. Because of the high incidence of recurrence and progression, elective endourologic management for grade III T1 tumors is not recommended. Some controversy still exists regarding the use of endoscopic management in patients with a normal contralateral kidney, in those who have multiple tumors in the same kidney or ipsilateral collecting system, and in patients with a solitary kidney with high-grade disease. This chapter describes the technique and discusses results of recent studies on percutaneous management of UTTCC. Recent results of instillation immuno- and chemotherapy for upper tract urothelial carcinoma are also discussed.

Keywords. Transitional cell, Upper urinary tract, Percutaneous, Ureter, Kidney

Introduction

The traditional treatment for upper tract urothelial carcinoma has been total nephroureterectomy with excision of a cuff of bladder tissue surrounding the ureteral orifice [1]. During the past two decades, numerous series on conserva-

---

[1]Department of Urology, Long Island Jewish Medical Center, New Hyde Park, NY 11040–1496, USA
[2]Division of Urology, University of Texas Health Science Center, San Antonio, TX, USA

tive surgery for renal pelvic and ureteral tumors reported acceptable outcomes in highly selected cases. In 1985, Huffman and colleagues reported the first truly endoscopic treatment of renal pelvic cancer using a transurethral ureteroscopic approach [2].

In 1986, Streem and Pontes reported the first percutaneous nephroscopic resection of upper tract tumors. This technique was subsequently popularized by Smith and colleagues [3,4]. The latter group also was the first to systematically instill antineoplastic agents into the renal pelvis percutaneously, based on prior anecdotal reports of topical thiotepa and bacillus Calmette–Guerin (BCG) administered in the ureter and kidney [5,6]. Laparoscopic nephroureterectomy, first described by Clayman and coworkers in 1991, provides a less invasive option for the removal of the entire kidney and ureter in patients requiring formal nephroureterectomy [7].

Development and refinement of endoscopic techniques, namely, percutaneous renal surgery, ureteroscopy, and laparoscopy, has enabled urologists to approach upper tract transitional cell carcinoma (UTTCC) in a less invasive fashion. Large tumors throughout the intrarenal collecting system can be approached using percutaneous tumor resection, while ureteral tumors are treated using ureteroscopy. The development of small flexible fiberoptic endoscopes has given the urologist retrograde access to the entire upper urinary tract. Ureteroscopy, thus, has been effective both diagnostically and therapeutically in the treatment of ureteral and renal transitional cell carcinoma (TCC). Finally, in those patients selected to undergo a formal nephroureterectomy, laparoscopy now provides an alternative to the open approach.

The rationale of treating urothelial cancers of the upper urinary tract by an endoscopic approach arose out of the need for renal preservation in some patients, as well as a desire to provide a less invasive and less morbid form of therapy wherever possible. However, endoscopic surgical techniques have not changed the basic tenet of solid tumor therapy, namely, complete extirpation of neoplastic tissue.

Today, endoscopic management is standard of care for patients with TCC in an anatomic or functional solitary kidney, patients with bilateral disease, and patients who are not candidates for open surgery due to underlying comorbidity, as long as they have noninvasive disease. However, controversy still exists regarding the use of endoscopic management in patients with a normal contralateral kidney, in those who have multiple tumors in the same kidney or ipsilateral collecting system, and in patients with a solitary kidney with high-grade disease.

Endoscopic surgery for upper tract carcinomas may also be indicated in patients with small grade 1, and to some extent grade 2, lesions. However, such patients must be willing to undergo rigorous post-treatment surveillance. High-grade (grade 3 or 4) lesions and tumors that appear to be invasive on radiographic imaging or direct endoscopic inspection should not be treated endoscopically in the presence of a normal contralateral kidney. Recurrence of a previously resected tumor to a higher grade or a tumor that recurs rapidly after resection and adjuvant therapy portends aggressive disease, and further attempts at endoscopic therapy are ill advised. Patients with active infection, bleeding diathesis or coagulopathy, and uncontrolled hypertension, which may increase the risk of postoperative hemorrhage, should not undergo endoscopic resection of upper tract urothelial carcinoma. Lastly, patients who are unable or unwilling to continue with a strict follow-up protocol should be excluded from definitive endoscopic therapy.

General Approach

Upper tract TCC most commonly presents with gross or microscopic hematuria, and subsequent workup with intravenous urography (IVU) or a computed tomography (CT) scan with contrast reveals a filling defect in the involved kidney or ureter. Positive urine cytology is highly suggestive of the diagnosis in the presence of an upper tract filling defect. In the absence of a visible lesion on urography, positive cytology from the upper tract may be indicative of carcinoma in situ and mandates ureteroscopic inspection of the kidneys and ureters. Figure 1 summarizes the management approach to UTTCC followed at Long Island Jewish Medical Center.

A CT scan before and after the administration of intravenous contrast is obtained to assess for evidence of parenchymal invasion. Computed tomography has the added benefits of excluding radiolucent stone as the cause of the filling defect, as well as ruling out the presence of gross abdominal metastases. If obvious invasion is noted on CT, a metastatic workup is performed (chest radiograph, liver function tests, bone scintigraphy), and the patient is directed toward laparoscopic nephroureterectomy. If CT fails to demonstrate parenchymal invasion, ureteropyeloscopy should be performed in order to verify the presence of TCC and to obtain a specimen for diagnostic, grading, and staging purposes. At the time of ureteroscopy, an attempt is made to completely resect the tumor. If the tumor is deemed unresectable due to size or poor visualization from bleeding, the patient undergoes a percutaneous resection. This can be done under the same anesthetic if the patient has been counseled about, and has consented to, this approach. If the ureteroscopic resection is adequate, a second-look ureteroscopy and biopsy is performed within 2–4 weeks to exclude residual disease. If this is negative, consideration is given to offering the patient adjuvant therapy with percutaneous instillation of BCG. If the tumor is still present on second-look ureteroscopy, this is resected and a final ureteroscopy is performed to assess the adequacy of treatment. Should the tumor persist at this time, the patient undergoes percutaneous resection, followed by a second-look nephroscopy within 1 week. If this is positive, the patient undergoes nephroureterectomy. If negative, the patient is given adjuvant BCG once per week for 6 weeks. A “third-look” nephroscopy and biopsy is performed 2 weeks after BCG therapy to exclude residual disease. A biopsy is necessary due to the

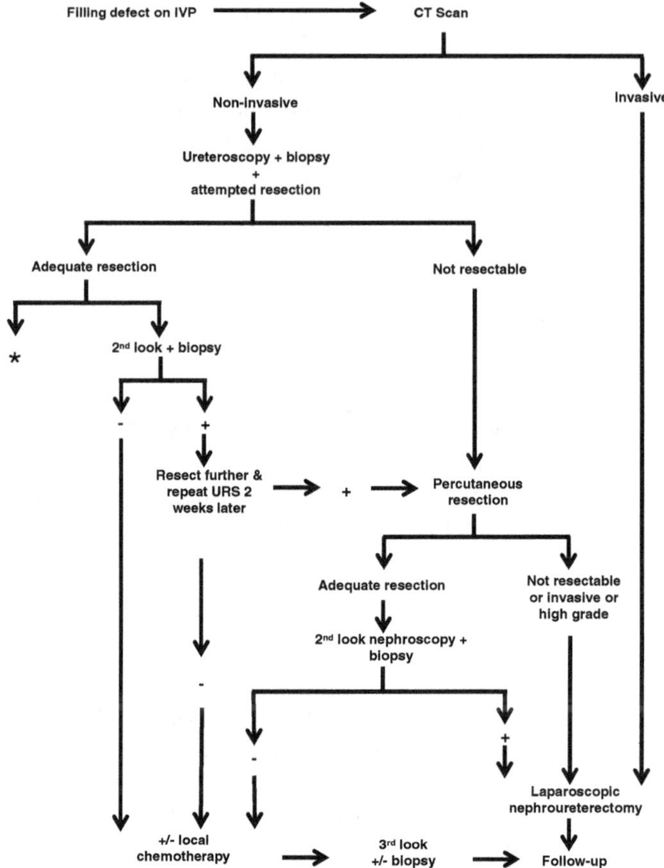

FIG. 1. Management approach to upper tract transitional cell carcinoma followed at Long Island Jewish Medical Center

difficulty of identifying residual tumor because of the inflammatory response induced by BCG and the presence of the nephrostomy tube.

Indications for Percutaneous Approach

Development of endoscopic techniques has enabled urologists to approach superficial UTTCC in a less invasive fashion. The main indication for an endoscopic approach is to preserve functional renal tissue. Patients with bulky and or low-grade (G1–G2) UTTCC limited to the renal pelvis who do not command a nephron-sparing approach may choose a percutaneous approach if appropriately counseled on the 25%–28% recurrence rate and the 5-year disease-specific survival of greater than 95%. Such patients must be motivated and reliable, as they will be subjected to a lifetime of endoscopic and radiographic surveillance. More commonly, conservative surgery for UTTCC is utilized in patients with bilateral synchronous tumors, cancer in a solitary kidney, and in patients with poor renal function in whom nephrectomy would result in the need for hemodialysis. Endoscopic surgery for UTTCC is reasonable as well in those patients with favorable tumor characteristics.

Contraindications to Percutaneous Approach

Biopsy proven high-grade (G3–G4) tumors and those appearing to be invasive on radiographic studies or endoscopic inspection should not be treated endoscopically in the presence of a normal contralateral kidney. If disease is unresectable due to size, number, or location of tumors, the patient should go on to a laparoscopic nephroureterectomy. If a previously resected lesion progresses to a higher grade or if a tumor recurs rapidly after resection and adjuvant instillation therapy, further attempts at primary endoscopic therapy should be abandoned.

Presence of an active infection, bleeding diathesis or coagulopathy, or uncontrolled hypertension should delay endoscopic resection until remedied. While morbid obesity is not a contraindication to a percutaneous approach, extra-long instruments may be needed to reach the kidney percutaneously; in such cases a ureteroscopic approach, if feasible, might be more effective.

Percutaneous Versus Ureteroscopic Approach

Both ureteroscopic and percutaneous approaches can be effective in the treatment of superficial TCC of the upper urinary tract, but each has certain advantages and disadvantages. Ureteroscopy is less invasive, relatively easy to perform, and imparts little risk of tumor spillage into the retroperitoneum. It is the best initial method for procuring a tissue sample adequate for diagnosis and grading, and it is the most thorough way to survey the whole collecting system during post-treatment follow-up. Ureteroscopy is the best approach for small lesions of the ureter or renal pelvis and obviates the risk of parenchymal hemorrhage or adjacent organ injury.

The main advantage of the percutaneous approach is that it allows the use of larger endoscopes, which improve visualization. The larger instruments used percutaneously facilitate resection of more extensive lesions and make tumor removal more efficient. Both rigid and flexible endoscopes may be passed through the percutaneous tract, so that all calices may be completely inspected. If a single tract is inadequate to reach all portions of the intrarenal collecting system, additional tracts can be created. A percutaneous approach may be the best choice for lower caliceal tumors that may not be accessible by ureteroscopy due to limitations in scope deflection. In patients with a prior urinary diversion, the percutaneous approach may be the only way to access the collecting system.

An impressive array of instruments can be used percutaneously, including larger resectoscopes and grasping and biopsy forceps, as well as larger-bore laser fibers. All tissue layers can be sampled percutaneously, potentially improving local tumor staging over ureteroscopy. Second look nephroscopy, biopsy, and, if necessary, residual tumor resection, are all facilitated by a percutaneous approach, as is the adjuvant instillation of BCG or mitomycin. However, the increased versatility of the percutaneous approach comes at the expense of greater morbidity compared to ureteroscopy, especially with regard to bleeding and the potential for adjacent organ injury.

Because of their distinct advantages, ureteroscopy and percutaneous resection should be thought of not as competing modalities, but complementary methods to accomplish the goal of complete tumor removal. Depending on tumor and patient characteristics, the management approach to UTTCC may encompass both treatments in an attempt to provide patients with the best quality in terms of diagnosis, therapy, and follow-up.

Patient Counseling

Patients who are candidates for an endoscopic approach by virtue of their tumor characteristics or because of impaired renal function must still be counseled that nephroureterectomy remains the gold standard treatment for UTTCC. They should understand that although their particular situation may warrant an endoscopic approach in order to spare renal function, they may at some later date require removal of the affected kidney entirely. On the other hand, patients with a solitary kidney or very poor renal function who are over the age of 65 years, should know that 5-year survival rates for elderly patients on dialysis are dismal, and that endoscopic management may afford them several years free of dialysis, with a potentially better quality of life.

Patients with a normal contralateral kidney who elect a conservative endoscopic approach must be made especially aware that this course of therapy imparts a higher risk of recurrence than nephroureterectomy, that progression to a higher grade or degree of invasion may occur, and that they may one day eventually lose the kidney. They should know that incidence of metachronous bilateral tumors is very low, only 1%–2% [8], and that this is less than the incidence of ipsilateral recurrence after percutaneous resection of even well-differentiated tumors [9]. It should also be made clear that there is little risk of developing renal insufficiency or hypertension, even years after removal of the diseased kidney [10]. Finally, patients must be willing to submit to an intense follow-up regimen which, because it includes frequent ureteroscopy, is more invasive and more expensive than the standard regimen following nephroureterectomy. Despite these caveats, patients should also understand that with favorable disease, there is a high likelihood of renal preservation.

In addition, the urologist should counsel the patient regarding the risks of the percutaneous approach itself, including bleeding necessitating blood transfusion, infection, failed access, injury to adjacent organs, and pleural injury. This discussion should be balanced by a discussion of the risks of open surgery as well as laparoscopic nephroureterectomy.

Ultimately, it is for the well-informed patient, taking into account his or her particular situation and the various risks and benefits, to come to a final decision about the choice of treatment approach.

Technique

Percutaneous surgery requires careful patient preparation. Since endoscopic management is indicated only for localized superficial disease, a metastatic work-up should be performed before resection is undertaken. This includes an abdominopelvic CT scan, chest X-ray, liver function tests, and serum alkaline phosphatase level. If the latter is elevated, bone scintigraphy is warranted.

To minimize the risk of bleeding and infection, anticoagulants should be stopped well in advance of surgery. Bleeding diathesis, active infection, and hypertension should be corrected or controlled before bringing the patient to the operating room. A positive urine culture is an absolute contraindication to proceed with percutaneous surgery and prolonged closed upper tract system manipulation.

The patient is given a first- or second-generation cephalosporin intravenously prior to surgery. Patients requiring prophylaxis against spontaneous bacterial endocarditis are given ampicillin and gentamicin, with vancomycin substituted if there is a penicillin allergy. Sequential compression devices are placed on both lower extremities to prevent deep vein thrombosis.

Cystoscopy is performed initially to rule out the presence of synchronous bladder tumor(s). A 5- or 6-F ureteral catheter is advanced into the renal pelvis. The ureteral catheter is fastened to a Foley catheter with a silk tie and the patient is then carefully transferred to the prone position. The face is padded with foam and chest bolsters are placed. The head and upper body padding should be adjusted so that the neck is in a neutral position. The elbows and knees are cushioned with foam or gel pads and the ankles are elevated on a bolster to prevent the toes from touching the table. The shoulders should be abducted to an angle of less than 90°. In morbidly obese patients, chest bolsters can be omitted.

Contrast is injected through the ureteral catheter to outline the pelvocaliceal system. To facilitate complete resection, caliceal tumors should be accessed with a puncture directly into the calix, while a pelvic tumor should be accessed through an upper or middle calix. While lower pole access to renal pelvic tumors has also been recommended [11], upper pole or middle caliceal access facilitates complete inspection of the collecting system with rigid endoscopes. With lower pole access, it may be impossible to pass a rigid scope into upper calices because the patient's hip can limit scope mobility.

After the access site is chosen, an 18-gauge diamond-tipped needle is passed into the collecting system under biplanar fluoroscopic guidance. The obturator is removed and efflux of urine confirms correct positioning of the needle. A guidewire is coiled in the collecting system or, preferably, advanced down the ureter. A second (safety) wire should be placed to guard against loss of the tract. The tract is created using a dilating balloon or sequential Amplatz dilators, and a working sheath is placed. To decrease the theoretical risk of tumor seeding, care should be taken to ensure that the sheath never slips out of the collecting system.

After dilation, nephroscopy of the entire system is carried out to identify all areas of tumor. If a guidewire cannot be manipulated down to the bladder, the tip of the ureteral catheter is grasped, pulled out through the nephrostomy, and intubated with a guidewire. The guidewire is then passed down to give through-and-through access. The safest way to excise the tumor is by piecemeal removal with cold-cup forceps. Biopsies of the tumor base are taken separately and then the base is resected and cauterized with a resectoscope or laser. Deep biopsies or resection into the renal parenchyma will result in a great deal of bleeding and should be avoided. If the operative field is clear enough, a flexible endoscope may be used to inspect the rest of the collecting system or address tumors that cannot be accessed with rigid instrumentation. At the conclusion of the operation, a 24-F Malecot nephrostomy tube with a ureteral extension is placed and its position verified under fluoroscopy. This large-bore catheter will tamponade parenchymal bleeding, provide excellent renal drainage, and preserve access to the kidney and ureter for the planned second-look nephroscopy.

Second-look nephroscopy is performed within 1 week of the initial resection, unless permanent section of the tumor reveals high-grade or invasive TCC, in which case nephroureterectomy is indicated. If the tumor is deemed not to be completely resectable through a percutaneous approach, a nephroureterectomy is done. The second look provides an opportunity to reinspect the urothelium in a relatively bloodless field, to excise any residual disease, and to biopsy the base of the previously resected tumor. High-grade or invasive disease on second-look biopsy is another indication for nephroureterectomy.

If intracavitary instillation of adjuvant agents is anticipated, the Malecot is exchanged for an 8-F pigtail nephrostomy catheter. Instillations may begin 2 weeks following the last resection. The authors have used mitomycin and BCG, but have more experience with the latter. The patient is admitted to the hospital for each BCG treatment or, alternatively, therapy may be undertaken in an outpatient chemotherapy infusion unit. Prophylactic intravenous antibiotics are mandatory because the nephrostomy tubes invariably become colonized and there is a risk of urosepsis. Fluoroquinolones, gentamicin, and doxycycline should *not* be used because they will inactivate the bacillus [12], but β-lactam antibiotics are acceptable. An infusion of normal saline into the nephrostomy tube is begun at 10cc per hour and increased by 10cc/h every 15min, until the infusion rate reaches 50cc/h. The intrarenal pressure is closely monitored to ensure that it remains below 25cmH_2O (Fig. 2). If the patient tolerates the saline infusion

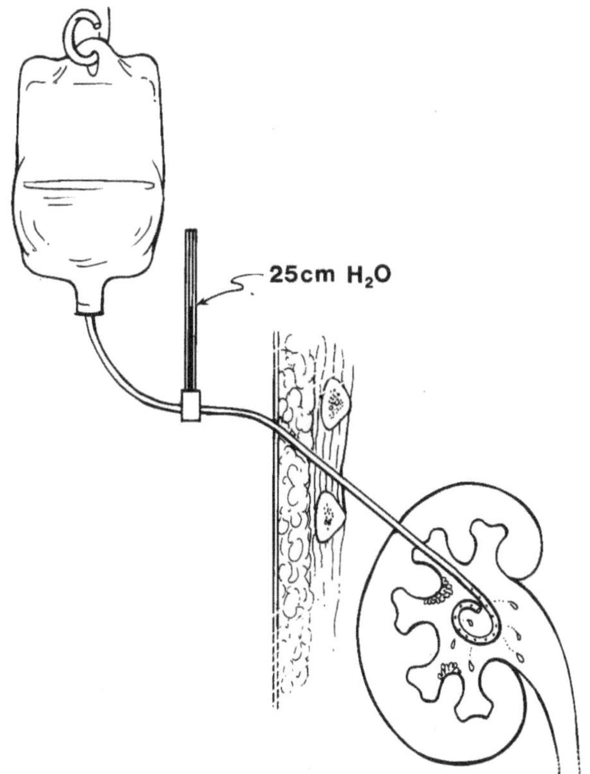

FIG. 2. Setup for intracavitary instillation of adjuvant agents into the upper collecting system for treatment of transitional cell carcinoma. The intrarenal pressure is closely monitored to ensure that it remains below 25 cmH_2O

without difficulty, 50 cc of 1×10^8 colony-forming units of BCG is administered over 1 h. The patient voids after instillation, and is discharged home the next day. Two weeks after completion of therapy, the patient undergoes a third-look nephroscopy, through the existing tract.

Results

There are few studies reporting the results of percutaneous management of UTTCC (Table 1), and three are from the same institution [9,13,14]. Almost all patients treated had solitary kidneys, bilateral disease, chronic renal failure, or significant comorbid disease contraindicating open surgery. At present, however, this is representative of the patient population most often considered for a percutaneous approach. Very few institutions have expanded the indications to

TABLE 1. Recurrence rates after percutaneous resection of upper tract transitional carcinoma, stratified by tumor grade

First author [Ref.]	Year	No. of patients	Follow-up (months)	Grade 1	Grade 2	Grade 3	Total
Plancke [19]	1995	10	28	1/6 (17%)	0/3	—	1/(911%)
Jarrett [9]	1995	34	56.4	2/11 (18%)	3/9 (33%)	5/10 (50%)	10/30 (33%)
Patel [18]	1996	26	44.7	2/11 (18%)	3/11 (27%)	—	6/25[a] (24%)
Clark [11]	1999	18	20.5	2/6 (13%)	2/8 (25%)	2/4 (50%)	6/18 (33%)
Lee [20]	1999	50	—	1/20 (5%)	1/16 (6%)	4/13 (31%)	6/49 (12%)
Jabbour [13]	2000	20	48	—	5/20 (25%)	—	5/20 (25%)
Liatsikos [14]	2001	69	49	3/15 (20%)	7/27 (26%)	14/25 (56%)	24/67 (36%)

[a]1/3 patients with unknown grade recurred.

include motivated, otherwise healthy patients, with superficial low-grade disease, who elect a nephron-sparing, minimally invasive approach [14–17]. Most recently, Palou et al. [16] presented their long-term data of percutaneous nephroscopic management of UTTCC in patients with papillary tumors of low grade and those lesions not amenable to ureteroscopic resection; grade III tumors were considered for resection only in those patients with a solitary kidney or bilateral disease. Almost half of these patients (44.1%, 16/34) were treated by a percutaneous route electively and all received adjuvant topical therapy with either BCG or mitomycin. Ipsilateral recurrence developed in 41.2% (14/34) of patients at a median time of 24 months.

Recurrence is the first measure of the efficacy of therapy, and tumor grade correlates well with recurrence (Table 1) [9,11,13,14,18–20]. It is clear that patients with grade 1 disease have a good prognosis, while outcomes of those with grade 3 tend to have a poorer response to treatment. Grade 1 disease recurs in 5%–33% of cases [9,11,14–20], but progression is less likely, and death from low-grade urothelial carcinoma is rare. There has been only one cancer-related death in a patient with grade 1 disease in four different series, and this patient was found to have grade 2 histology on second look [9,14,19,20]. Grade 1 lesions are associated with a good rate of renal preservation. Of 15 patients with grade 1 disease, only one underwent nephroureterectomy while the two other recurrences were treated endoscopically [14].

The prognosis of grade 2 disease is also good. Recurrence rate in 99 patients from seven different series is 21% [9,11,13,14,18–20]. In four of the five studies where disease-specific survival is reported or can be calculated, patients with grade 2 pathology died of cancer-related causes in less than 5% of cases. Renal retention, however, is a serious consideration. Jarrett et al. reported that of 12 patients with grade 2 histology, six (50%) required nephroureterectomy, three within days of their percutaneous resection, and three for recurrence [9]. Jabbour and associates published a study that specifically addressed grade 2 disease managed with percutaneous resection. They found that seven of 24 patients (29%) underwent nephroureterectomy, four immediately and three for recurrence [13].

The prognosis for high-grade UTTCC is poor, regardless of management modality. In the largest published series of grade 3 patients, Liatsikos and colleagues reported 56% recurrence and 64% disease-specific survival [14]. Jarrett and associates included 13 grade 3 patients in their series. Eight of them died during follow-up, six of disease-related causes (46%), and of those without evidence of disease, only one patient had retained the affected kidney [9]. The disparity between the two studies may be explained by the shorter follow-up time in the report by Liatsikos et al. It is evident that percutaneous resection should not be offered for high-grade UTTCC, except as a last resort in elderly patients with a solitary kidney, who would not tolerate hemodialysis.

Tumor stage also imparts prognosis in association with grade. Noninvasive (Ta) lesions generally tend to be low grade. In one study, all patients with grade 1 lesions had Ta disease [9], while in the studies of Plancke et al. [19] and Martinez-Pineiro et al. [21], Ta was seen in 86% and 76% of grade 1 tumors, respectively [19,21]. Superficially invasive (T1) tumors tend to be more heter ogeneous, with substantial numbers of these lesions occurring as grade 2 and 3 disease [9,21].

The effect of stage on recurrence and disease-free survival can be seen in a study by Jabbour and associates, in which 54 patients were followed for a mean of 50 months after percutaneous resection of UTTCC. Stage Ta was associated with 30% recurrence and 93% disease-free survival, while T1 tumors recurred 57% of the time and were associated with 64% disease-free survival. Stage retained its prognostic significance when stratified by grade [22]. The poorer prognosis of the higher stage has been confirmed by other investigators. Patel and coworkers found that T1 had a higher recurrence rate than Ta (30% vs. 12.5%) [18], and Jarrett and associates found worse disease-specific survival (92% vs. 57%) [9].

A final consideration is the risk of disease recurrence in the percutaneous tract, which was initially thought to be a significant hazard due to the potential of tumor seeding the tract. Irradiation of the tract was used in two studies in order to avoid seeding in patients treated percutaneously [18,23]. While no cases of tract recurrence occurred in either of these reports, most institutions offering a percutaneous approach have not employed tract irradiation and, in the majority, no cases of tract seeding have been encountered [9,11,13–15,18–22].

There have been three case reports of tract seeding occurring in situations that were not typical of current treatment protocols [23–25]. In one case, due to delay in diagnosis of the etiology of a ureteral obstruction, the percutaneous tract was exposed to high-grade TCC for 1 month prior to resection; while in the other, a second-look procedure to rule out persistence of unresected disease was never undertaken. These two examples highlight the importance of complete tumor resection, second- and third-look nephroscopy and biopsy to ensure that no disease is left behind, and minimizing the time that the tract is exposed to unresected cancer. Thirdly, and most recently, Oefelein and MacLennan reported on a TCC nephrostomy tract recurrence following percutaneous resection of a T1G2 lesion in a patient who had undergone prior radical cystectomy for T2N0M0 disease [25]. The patient eventually underwent a nephroureterectomy with upstaging to T2N1M0 disease status. Four months postoperatively, a TCC nephrostomy tract recurrence presented as an erythematous papule. Despite tract excision, local radiation, and chemotherapy, the patient soon died of metastatic TCC. Although this mortality was associated with a TCC nephrostomy tract recurrence, it is more likely that the patient succumbed to his disease as a result of nodal involvement.

Considerable experience demonstrates that the risk of tumor seeding in appropriately selected patients is negligible. A recent study by Czito et al. investigated the role of adjuvant radiotherapy with and without concurrent chemotherapy for locally advanced TCC of the renal pelvis and ureter [26]. Findings in this report suggest that the addition of concurrent cisplatin to adjuvant radiotherapy improves the ultimate outcome in patients with resected, locally advanced upper tract urothelial malignancies. Although this study was in a cohort of patients who underwent extirpative rather than endoscopic treatment, perhaps such findings suggest a future role for adjuvant or neoadjuvant treatments involving endoscopic resection for high-grade disease.

Complications of Percutaneous Resection

Percutaneous resection of UTTCC can generally be accomplished safely. Bleeding requiring transfusion occurs in 11%–37% of cases [11,15,18,22], and can result from injury to a vessel during creation of the percutaneous tract, or it may be due to the resection itself. If bleeding during establishment of the tract is so brisk as to impair visualization, the procedure should be abandoned. Tamponade of the tract with a large-bore nephrostomy tube or a Kaye balloon catheter will usually limit bleeding in such situations and the procedure can be resumed in 2–3 days. Angiography with super-selective embolization is reserved for those cases in which such conservative measures fail to adequately control hemorrhage.

In contrast to bleeding from the nephrostomy tract, hemorrhage occurring as a result of tumor resection is effectively controlled only by complete tumor resection or fulguration. Factors influencing the degree of blood loss include the grade and size of the tumor, as well as the depth of resection [22]. It is important to avoid resecting too deeply into parenchyma, as this will greatly increase the risk of bleeding. Complete resection of invasive disease is dangerous as well as unnecessary, since this situation is best treated by nephroureterectomy. Use of a vaporization electrode or Nd:YAG laser to fulgurate the tumor base may help to reduce the occurrence of significant bleeding [22].

Perforation of the renal pelvis should be avoided because of the potential for tumor spill into the retroperitoneum, although no such cases have been reported. Since tumor resection cannot be performed with saline irrigation, extravasation of fluid into the retroperitoneum may lead to hyponatremia. Recognition of a significant tear in the collecting system during resection mandates expedient completion of the procedure and placement of a large-bore nephrostomy tube to facilitate drainage and resolution of the defect.

Other potential complications are related to percutaneous renal surgery in general and include fever, urinary tract infection, failure to obtain access, and injury to adjacent structures such as pleura or bowel. Fever occurs in 5%–10% of cases [11,15], while the others are much less common.

Strictures of the infundibulum or ureteropelvic junction may occur as late complications. These should be investigated by direct visualization with ureteroscopy and possible biopsy to rule out recurrent tumor as the etiology. Such strictures occurred in 8.7% of cases in one study of 23 patients [21]. They can be managed ureteroscopically or by percutaneous infundibulotomy or endopyelotomy.

Surveillance for Percutaneous and Ureteroscopic Resection

Lifelong surveillance is an absolute requisite for those patients treated primarily with endoscopic resection because of the potential for recurrence. Since most recurrences occur within 3 years of initial therapy [27], the follow-up regimen may be tailored to this pattern.

Due to the 30%–70% risk of recurrent bladder TCC in those with previous upper tract disease, cystoscopy should be performed every 3 months for 1 year, biannually during the second year, and then yearly thereafter. Surveillance ureteroscopy is the modality of choice to follow the upper tracts due to the lack of sensitivity of excretory urography and retrograde pyelography. Chen and associates found the sensitivity of ureteroscopy with biopsy was 93.4% compared with 71.7% for retrograde pyelography [28], while Keeley and coworkers diagnosed only one fourth of recurrences by retrograde pyelography alone [29]. A reasonable surveillance regimen for the upper tract involves uretereroscopy at 6-month intervals for the first 3 years and then annually thereafter. The contralateral kidney, if present, should be imaged annually with either retrograde or excretory pyelography.

Instillation Therapy in Upper Tract Urothelial Carcinoma

In 1985, Herr reported a case of a patient with a solitary kidney who had been treated for muscle invasive urothelial carcinoma with wide excision of the renal pelvis and entire ureter followed by creation of a pyelovesical anastomosis. The margins of the resected pelvis and infundibula were positive for carcinoma in situ, so the patient underwent a 6-week course of BCG instillation via the bladder. The patient's urinary cytology normalized and remained negative for over 13 months [30]. In 1986, Streem and Pontes reported on a patient with urothelial carcinoma of a solitary kidney treated with percutaneous resection followed by adjuvant mitomycin C [3]. The following year, Smith and coworkers published results on a series of nine patients treated with percutaneous resection; five of these patients received adjuvant BCG [4]. Since that time, a number of institutions have reported the use of instillation therapy with BCG, mitomycin, epirubicin, or thiotepa, either as primary treatment for carcinoma in situ or as adjuvant therapy after resection or ablation of papillary tumors. Currently, BCG is the most commonly used agent.

Topical immuno- or chemotherapy delivery may be accomplished by retrograde instillation through a ureteral catheter, via vesicoureteral reflux from an indwelling ureteral stent, or through a pigtail nephrostomy tube. The disadvantage of retrograde catheterization is that cystoscopy must be performed prior to each instillation. To overcome this, Patel and Fuchs passing a single-J ureteral stent through a percutaneous cystotomy and securing it to the skin of the abdomen, obviating the need for endoscopy prior to each instillation [31]. The retrograde techniques may be more expedient when the initial resection is performed ureteroscopically or when instillation is done as primary therapy for CIS—situations in which a nephrostomy tube is not routinely used. Others have advocated a pigtail nephrostomy tube for all instillations, even those in which percutaneous resection is not required, speculating that contact of the agent with the urothelium is maximized by antegrade administration [32]. A potential disadvantage of the reflux technique is the uncertainty of how much agent actually reaches the renal collecting system. Irie and colleagues performed cystograms to determine the amount of fluid required to induce reflux in each of their patients after placement of a double-J stent. This volume, which ranged from 80 to 250cc, was used to guide the subsequent instillation volume of BCG [33]. Another disadvantage of the retrograde technique is infusion of a drug into a system that is obstructed by a ureteral catheter, which increases the risk of Gram-negative sepsis and BCG absorption. To lessen this risk, it would be prudent to perform infusion of the drug through a double-lumen catheter. The main critique of percutaneous instillation is the potential for tumor seeding of the nephrostomy tract during the 6 or more weeks that the tube is in place; however, current protocols emphasize the need for second-look nephroscopy and biopsy to exclude persistence of tumor prior to undertaking instillation therapy. While each method has pros and cons, no evidence in the literature favors any one technique over another.

BCG immunotherapy may be used as primary treatment for upper tract carcinoma in situ. Positive initial response rates range from 60% to 100%, with an overall response rate of 84% (Table 2) [33–39]. These data, however, are based on normalization of selective urinary cytology, a far less rigorous criterion for success than ureteroscopy and biopsy. Of the initial responders in these studies, one fourth experienced an upper tract recurrence and almost 10% eventually

TABLE 2. Positive response and local recurrence rates after primary therapy of upper tract carcinoma-in-situ with bacillus Calmette–Guerin

First author [Ref.]	Year	No. of patients	Positive response	Upper tract recurrence
Sharpe [34]	1993	11	8 (73%)	0/8
Yokogi [35]	1996	5	3 (60%)	0/3
Nishino [36]	2000	6	6 (100%)	0/6
Nonomura [37]	2000	11	9 (82%)	2/9 (22%)
Okubo [38]	2001	11	8 (73%)	3/8 (37%)
Irie [33]	2002	9	9 (100%)	0/9
Thalmann [39]	2002	21	19 (90%)	11/19 (58%)
Total		74	62 (84%)	16/62 (26%)

TABLE 3. Local recurrence rates for upper tract transitional carcinoma treated by primary percutaneous or endoscopic resection followed by adjuvant bacillus Calmette–Guerin

First author [Ref.]	Year	No. of patients	Upper tract recurrence
Schoenberg [41]	1991	9	1 (11%)
Martinez-Pineiro [21]	1996	8	1 (12.5%)
Patel [31]	1998	12	2 (16.7%)
Clark [11]	1999	18	6 (33%)
Jabbour [22]	2000	30	9 (30%)
Thalmann [39]	2002	14	12 (85.7%)
Total		91	31 (34%)

developed metastatic disease. Fifteen percent died of urothelial carcinoma and 13.5% died of other causes within an overall mean follow-up period of 35 months [40].

A beneficial role for topical adjuvant therapy following resection of papillary upper tract tumors has not been proven. No randomized trials of adjuvant therapy have been performed, due to the relative rarity of UTTCC. Even a multi-institutional effort would take years to reach any conclusions; however, such a trial would be useful in guiding therapy. Currently, six series specifically assessing adjuvant BCG exist (Table 3) [11,21,22,31,39,41]. Recurrence rates range from 11% to 85%, although they are closer to 30% in the two largest series. Stratification by grade yields recurrence rates of 17% for grade 1, 20% for grade 2, and 44% for grade 3, from 76 total patients. These rates do not include the study by Thalmann and associates, which had the highest overall recurrence (85%) [39], because this study did not stratify recurrence by grade. To date there has been only one report comparing outcomes of patients who received postresection BCG versus those who did not, and it failed to show any benefit for grade 2 or 3 disease. However, there was a significantly lower recurrence rate in grade 1 patients receiving BCG compared with those who got no adjuvant therapy [22].

In addition to not being randomized, this analysis lacked sufficient power to definitively exclude an advantage for the higher grades.

The use of adjuvant therapy in grade 2 or 3 disease, despite lack of strong evidence to support the practice, is attractive because of its potential benefits and its relative safety when administered with the appropriate precautions outlined previously. Furthermore, several factors, including the well-known increased risk of recurrence with medium- or high-grade disease in the face of an anatomic or functional solitary kidney, as well as the risk and invasiveness of treating recurrences in patients with normal renal function, serve as an impetus to do as much as possible with adjuvant therapy.

The major complications of upper tract BCG instillation are BCG dissemination and urosepsis secondary to Gram-negative organisms, with both of these being relatively rare occurrences. In one series of 11 patients there was one case of BCG dissemination [34]. Another study reported two patients with sepsis and one with BCG dissemination out of 37 patients treated [39]. Minor complications such as fever without infection and the presence of irritative voiding symptoms throughout the treatment period are more common. Fever has been reported in up to 67% of patients in one series [36], and colonization of the nephrostomy tube with skin flora is frequent. Biopsies during post-BCG nephroscopy may reveal renal granulomata, but these generally have no clinical significance [42].

Conclusion

Percutaneous management of UTTCC is indicated and ideal for addressing bulky low-grade papillary TCC limited to the renal calices, pelvis, or proximal ureter. Ureteroscopy may be utilized initially to treat papillary lesions anywhere along the upper tract urothelium as long as it is technically feasible. Due to technological advancements and refinement in endoscopic technique, most patients with UTTCC can now be offered minimally invasive treatment with either single- or multi-modal approaches involving ureteroscopy, percutaneous resection, or laparoscopic nephroureterectomy. A role for BCG in the treatment of upper tract carcinoma in situ has been demonstrated; however, definitive efficacy of adjuvant topical therapy following endoscopic resection of UTTCC has not been proven. In this regard, multi-institutional studies are called for. For those motivated patients with noninvasive, low-to-medium grade disease, endourologic therapy provides a reasonable treatment option. In those patients with a functional or solitary kidney, conservative endourologic management of even high-grade disease may delay the need for nephrectomy and renal replacement therapy. Long-term rigorous follow-up after endourologic treatment, especially with regular surveillance ureteroscopy, is critical to diagnose and treat recurrences in a timely manner and therefore maintain acceptable cancer-free survival rates.

References

1. Kimball FN, Ferris HW (1934) Papillomatous tumor of the renal pelvis associated with similar tumors of the ureter and bladder: review of the literature and report of two cases. J Urol 31:257–259
2. Huffman JL, Bagley DH, Lyon ES, Morse MJ, Herr HW, Whitmore WFJ (1985) Endoscopic diagnosis and treatment of upper tract urothelial tumors. A preliminary report. Cancer 55:1422–1428
3. Streem SB, Pontes EJ (1986) Percutaneous management of upper tract transitional cell carcinoma. J Urol 135:773–775
4. Smith AD, Orihuela E, Crowley AR (1987) Percutaneous management of renal pelvic tumors: treatment option in selected cases. J Urol 137:852–856
5. Herr HW (1985) Durable response of a carcinoma in situ of the renal pelvis to topical bacillus Calmette–Guerin. J Urol 134:531–532
6. Powder JR, Mosberg WH, Pierpoint RZ (1984) Bilateral primary carcinoma of the ureter: topical and: ureteral thiotepa. J Urol 132:349–352
7. Clayman RV, Kavoussi LR, Figenshau RS, Chandhoke PS, Albala DM (1991) Laparoscopic nephroureterectomy: initial clinical case report. J Laparoendosc Surg 1(6):343–349
8. Clayman RV, McDougall EM, Nakada SY (1998) Endourology of the upper urinary tract: percutaneous renal and ureteral procedures. In: Walsh PC, Retik AB, Vaughan ED, Wein AJ (eds) Campbell's urology, vol. 3. Saunders, Philadelphia, pp 2831–2836
9. Jarrett TW, Sweetser PM, Weiss GH, Smith AD (1995) Percutaneous management of transitional cell carcinoma of the renal collecting system: 9-year experience. J Urol 154:1629–1635
10. Wishnow KI, Johnson DE, Preston D, Tenney D (1990) Long-term serum creatinine values after radical nephrectomy. Urology 35:114–116
11. Clark PE, Streem SB, Geisinger MA (1999) 13-year experience with percutaneous management of upper tract transitional cell carcinoma. J Urol 161:772–776
12. Durek C, Rusch-Gerdes S, Jocham D, Bohle A (2000) Sensitivity of BCG to modern antibiotics. Eur Urol 37:21–25
13. Jabbour ME, Desgrandchamps F, Cazin S, Teillac P, Le Duc A, Smith AD (2000) Percutaneous management of grade II upper urinary tract transitional cell carcinoma: the long-term outcome. J Urol 163:1105–1107
14. Liatsikos EN, Dinlenc CZ, Kapoor R, Smith AD (2001) Transitional-cell carcinoma of the Renal Pelvis: Ureteroscopic and percutaneous approach. J Endourol 15(4): 377–383
15. Elliot DS, Segura JW, Lightner D, Patterson DE, Blute ML (2001) Is nephroureterectomy necessary in all cases of upper tract transitional carcinoma? Long-term results of conservative endourologic management of upper tract transitional cell carcinoma in individuals with a normal contralateral kidney. Urology 58:174–178
16. Palou J, Piovesan LF, Huguet J, Salvador J, Vincente J, Villavicencio H (2004) Percutaneous nephroscopic management of upper urinary tract transitional cell carcinoma: recurrence and long-term followup. J Urol 172:66–69
17. Goel MC, Mahendra V, Roberts JG (2003) Percutaneous management of renal pelvic urothelial tumors: long-term followup. J Urol 169:925–930
18. Patel A, Soonawalla P, Shepherd SF, Dearnaley DP, Kellett MJ, Woodhouse CRJ (1996) Long-term outcome after percutaneous treatment of transitional cell carcinoma of the renal pelvis. J Urol 155:868–874

19. Plancke HR, Strijbos WE, Delaere KP (1995) Percutaneous endoscopic treatment of urothelial tumours of the renal pelvis. Br J Urol 75:736–739
20. Lee BR, Jabbour ME, Marshall FF, Smith AD, Jarrett TW (1999) 13-year survival comparison of percutaneous and open nephroureterectomy approaches for management of transitional cell carcinoma of renal collecting system: Equivalent outcomes. J Endourol 13:289–294
21. Martinez-Pineiro JA, Matres Garcia MJ, Martinez-Pineiro L (1996) Endourological treatment of upper tract urothelial carcinomas: analysis of a series of 59 tumors. J Urol 156:377–385
22. Jabbour ME, Smith AD (2000) Primary percutaneous approach to upper urinary tract transitional cell carcinoma. Urol Clin North Am 27:739–750
23. Sharma NK, Nicol A, Powell CS (1994) Tract infiltration following percutaneous resection of renal pelvic transitional cell carcinoma. Br J Urol 73:597–598
24. Huang A, Low RK, White R (1995) Case reports: Nephrostomy tract tumor seeding following percutaneous manipulation of a ureteral carcinoma. J Urol 153:1041–1042
25. Oefelein MG, MacLennan G (2003) Transitional cell carcinoma recurrence in the nephrostomy tract after percutaneous resection. J Urol 170:521
26. Czito B, Zietman A, Kaufman D, Skowronski U, Shipley W (2004) Adjuvant radiotherapy with and without concurrent chemotherapy for locally advanced transitional cell carcinoma of the renal pelvis and ureter. J Urol 172:1271–1275
27. Mills IW, Laniado ME, Patel A (2001) The role of endoscopy in the management of patients with upper urinary tract transitional cell carcinoma. BJU Int 87:150–162
28. Chen GL, El-Gabry EA, Bagley DH (2000) Surveillance of upper urinary tract transitional cell carcinoma: the role of ureteroscopy, retrograde pyelography, cytology and urinalysis. J Urol 165:1901–1904
29. Keeley FX, Bibbo M, Bagley DH (1997) Ureteroscopic treatment and surveillance of upper urinary tract transitional cell carcinoma. J Urol 157: 1560–1565
30. Herr HW(1985) Durable response of a carcinoma in situ of the renal pelvis to topical bacillus Calmette–Guerin. J Urol 134:531–532
31. Patel A, Fuchs GJ (1998) New techniques for the administration of topical adjuvant therapy after endoscopic ablation of upper urinary tract transitional cell carcinoma. J Urol 159:71–75
32. Studer UE, Casanova G, Kraft R, Zingg EJ (1989) Percutaneous bacillus Calmette–Guerin perfusion of the upper urinary tract for carcinoma in situ. J Urol 142:975–977
33. Irie A, Iwamura M, Kadowaki K, Ohkawa A, Uchida T, Baba S (2002) Intravesical instillation of bacillus Calmette–Guerin for carcinoma in situ of the urothelium involving the upper urinary tract utilizing vesicoureteral reflux created by a double-pigtail catheter. Urology 59:53–57
34. Sharpe JR, Duffy G, Chin JL (1993) Intrarenal bacillus Calmette–Guerin therapy for upper urinary tract carcinoma in situ. J Urol 149:457–460
35. Yokogi H, Wada Y, Mizutani M, Igawa M, Ishibe T (1996) Bacillus Calmette Guerin perfusion therapy for carcinoma in situ of the upper urinary tract. Br J Urol 77:676–679
36. Nishino Y, Yamammoto N, Komeda H, Takahashi Y, Deguchi T (2000) Bacillus Calmette–Guerin instillation treatment for carcinoma in situ of the upper urinary tract. BJU Int 85:799–801
37. Nonomura N, Ono Y, Nozawa M, Fukui T, Harada Y, Nishimura K, Takaha N, Takahara S, Okuyama A (2000) Bacillus Calmette–Guerin perfusion therapy for the

treatment of transitional cell carcinoma in situ of the upper urinary tract. Eur Urol 38:701–705
38. Okubo K, Ichioka K, Terada N, Matsuta Y, Arai YK (2001) Intrarenal bacillus Calmette–Guerin therapy for carcinoma in situ of the upper urinary tract: long-term follow-up and natural course in cases of failure. BJU Int 88:343–347
39. Thalmann GN, Markwalder R, Walter B, Studer UE (2002) Long term experience with bacillus Calmette–Guerin therapy of upper urinary tract transitional cell carcinoma in patients not eligible for surgery. J Urol 168:1381–1385
40. Marcovich R, Jacobson A, Smith A (2004). Percutaneous upper tract-preserving approaches in urothelial cancer. In: Droller MJ (ed) Treatment of upper tract urothelial cancer: American Cancer Society atlas of clinical oncology—urothelial tumors. Decker, Hamilton, pp 340–352
41. Schoenberg MP, Van Arsdalen KN, Wein AJ (1991) The management of transitional cell carcinoma in solitary renal units. J Urol 1991; 146:700–703
42. Bellman GC, Sweetser P, Smith D (1994) Complications of intracavitary bacillus Calmette–Guerin after percutaneous resection of upper tract transitional cell carcinoma. J Urol 151:13–15

Ureteroscopic Approach to Transitional Cell Carcinoma of the Upper Urinary Tract

Ioannis M. Varkarakis[1] and Thomas W. Jarrett[2]

Summary. In patients for whom renal sparing surgery is mandated secondary to a solitary kidney, renal insufficiency, bilateral disease, or high surgical risk, or patients with small, low-grade tumors, ureteroscopic management is evolving as an alternative to radical nephroureterectomy. Smaller rigid and flexible ureteroscopes have allowed for the detection and sampling of urothelial tumors located almost anywhere in the upper urinary tract. New laser technologies provide effective tumor ablation capabilities with low risk of complications. Long-term safety in properly selected patients has been proven in several studies. However, recurrences are expected and thus vigilant follow-up of the entire upper urinary tract and bladder is necessary. Adjuvant topical therapies appear to be safe but confirmation of any benefits awaits the results of further large studies.

Keywords. Transitional cell carcinoma, Ureteroscopy, Management

Introduction: Natural History of Upper Urinary Tract TCC and Indications for Conservative Therapy

Upper urinary tract urothelial tumors are rare, accounting for 1%–2% of all genitourinary tumors [1]. The vast majority are transitional cell carcinomas (TCC) (90%), while only 10% are squamous cell carcinomas and 1% adenocarcinomas [2]. Urothelial tumors of the ureter are 3–4 times less frequent than those located in the renal pelvis [3].

The incidence of upper urinary tract TCC increases with age in both sexes, and appears most frequently during the 6th and 7th decades of life. Males present with this disease 3 times more frequently than women [4].

[1] Second Department of Urology, University of Athens, 1 Sismanogliou Str, 15126, Marousi, Greece

[2] The James Buchanan Brady Urological Institute, Johns Hopkins Medical Institutions, 600 North Wolfe Street, Suite 161, Jefferson Street Bldg, Baltimore, MD 21287–8915, USA

Like that of the bladder, upper urinary tract TCC most likely represents a field change disease with multiple recurrences in both time and space. This polychronotropism is generally confined to the ipsilateral renal unit or to the bladder. While recurrence at an additional site in the genitourinary system will occur in 30%–50% of patients [5], recurrence in the contralateral renal unit will develop only in 1%–5.8% [6,7]. This natural history makes nephroureterectomy with resection of a bladder cuff safe and effective for therapy of an upper urinary tract TCC. Rates of local or ipsilateral recurrence after nephron-preserving surgery are high, and therefore conservative management with renal sparing procedures has been implemented only when preservation of renal function is necessary. This includes patients with an anatomically or functionally solitary kidney, those with bilateral disease, and patients who refuse or are unable to tolerate open surgery due to medical comorbidities (Table 1).

Recent advances in endoscopic technology with the development of better optics, actively deflecting telescopes, and adjunctive instrumentation allow us to diagnose and stage more accurately patients with upper urinary TCC. In fact, direct visualization of the tumor allows for a tumor biopsy and selective urine cytology to be done. Tumor grading in this setting is very accurate and is 90% in agreement with the grade of the final pathological specimen. In contrast, ureteroscopic biopsy is unreliable in determining stage [8]. However, several studies have suggested a good correlation between the grade of TCC and the stage of the tumor [9,10], and high accuracy of the computed tomography (CT) scan in detecting evidence of tumor extension beyond the wall of the ureter or renal pelvis [11]. Therefore the combination of low grade on biopsy, negative urine cytologies, and absence of frank extension outside of the urinary tract by CT scan strongly suggests the disease is superficial [12,13]. These criteria create a new subset of patients with small and low-grade tumors that can potentially be managed by endoscopic management only, even in the presence of a healthy contralateral kidney [14]. Although the cancer-related risks are greater for any treatment short of the gold standard nephroureterectomy, some patients are better treated by parenchymal-sparing surgery, provided they know the risks and are committed to vigilant follow-up.

Both ureteroscopic and percutaneous tumor resection are possible and are used in selected centers for up to 15% of patients with upper urinary TCC [15].

TABLE 1. Indications for ureteroscopic management of upper tract urothelial tumors

Indications for conservative therapy
Solitary kidney
Bilateral tumors
Limited renal function
Medical comorbidities preventing more invasive treatment
Low-grade, low-stage distal ureteral tumors

The approach selected depends largely on the tumor location and size. In general a retrograde ureteroscopic approach is used for low volume ureteral and renal tumor, while the antegrade percutaneous approach is chosen for larger tumors located proximally in the renal pelvis and or upper ureter, and those that can not be adequately manipulated in a retrograde approach owing to difficult location.

The main advantage of the ureteroscopic approach is its lesser invasiveness compared with the antegrade/percutaneous approach. In addition, the integrity of the collecting system is maintained throughout the procedure, thus diminishing the potential risk for transitional tumor cell spillage [16]. However, working channels in the ureteroscope are smaller than those of the nephroscope. Visualization is worse and the ability of resecting large tumor burdens decreases. Thus extensive resection similar to that performed in the bladder or the percutaneous approach is not possible. Similarly, staging biopsies during ureteroscopy are not as deep due to the risk of perforation and therefore may be less reliable in accurately staging the disease. Occasionally tumor location may preclude the ureteroscopic approach. However, a new generation of flexible ureteroscopes and small-diameter rigid ureteroscopes provide the ability to treat small endothelial tumors located even in the most challenging locations (e.g., lower pole calyx).

Instrumentation

- C-arm configuration fluoroscopy equipment
- Rigid cystoscope with working channel, 30° and 70° lenses
- Minor cystoscopy instruments
- Guide-wires: 0.025-inch straight Amplatz extra stiff or 0.038-inch straight heavy-duty Teflon or 0.038-inch hydrophilic coated, angled, and straight
- Balloon or other ureteral dilators
- Semi rigid ureteroscope
- Flexible ureteroscope
- Rigid ureteral resectoscope (12F)
- Biopsy forceps (3F)
- Flat wire baskets or grasping forceps
- Small electrocautery probe (2–3F)
- Ho:YAG or Nd:YAG laser with appropriate laser fibers
- Ureteral stents (self retaining double J, catheter 6F open ended, cone-tip catheter 8F, catheter 10F dual lumen)

Technique

Preoperative evaluation should include a coagulation profile with negative urine cultures.

After spinal or induction of general anesthesia, patients are placed in dorsal lithotomy position and are prepped and draped in the standard sterile fashion. Rigid cystoscopy is performed to confirm the absence of disease in the bladder and identify any lateralizing hematuria coming from the ureteral orifices. Retrograde pyelography may be done at the time of the procedure, if not recently performed during the diagnostic evaluation, in order to confirm exact tumor location.

Inspection of the lower and mid ureter is usually performed with rigid ureteroscopy. Small-diameter rigid ureteroscopes (6–10F) are typically used and usually do not require any active dilatation of the ureteral orifice. Larger rigid ureteroscopes have larger working channels and provide a wider field of view and better irrigation, but may require ureteral dilation.

A soft-tipped ureteral stent is then placed under fluoroscopic guidance up to the level of the tumor. An effort should be made not to pass the guide wire or the endoscope onto or beyond the level of the tumor in order to avoid bleeding, which in turn will obscure good visualization and make subsequent resection difficult. Stent placement facilitates ureteral navigation through proximal parts of the ureter with flexible ureteroscopy. Modern flexible ureteropyeloscopes are available in sizes smaller than 8F to allow for simple and reliable passage to most portions of the urinary tract, especially in the male patient [17,18]. However, flexible ureteroscopes have technical limitations, such as a small working channel that limits irrigant flow and the diameter of working instruments. Tumors in locations not amenable to the ureteroscopic approach should be dealt with in an antegrade fashion.

Once a suspicious lesion is detected, a normal saline wash of the area is performed before tumor biopsy or ablation [19]. Tumor sampling and biopsies are then performed with either a 2.5F flat wire basket or a 3F cup biopsy forceps. Regardless of the technique used, special attention to biopsy specimens is necessary. These specimens are frequently minute and should be placed in fixative at once and specially labeled for either histologic or cytologic evaluation [20]. Both the tumor and surrounding mucosa may be sampled to evaluate the extent of the disease and to rule out the possibility of carcinoma in situ. Extensive biopsies, however, may be difficult using smaller endoscopes.

Furthermore, grasping forceps or a flat wire basket may be used to debulk the tumor down to its base in a piecemeal fashion. The specimen is again sent for pathologic evaluation and the base of the tumor, after being biopsied, is subsequently ablated either with electrocautery or a form of laser energy. This technique is especially useful for papillary tumors on a thin stalk.

Alternatively the tumor may be resected to its base with a ureteroscopic resectoscope. Only the intraluminal tumor is resected, and no attempt is made to resect deep (beyond the lamina propria). Extra care is necessary in the mid and upper ureter, where the wall is quite thin and prone to perforation. Ureteral resectoscopes are approximately 12F and require active dilation of the ureteral orifice. Because of the relatively small capacity of the ureter, the specimen must be removed after each loop and irrigation drained in order to keep visualization optimal and prevent migration of specimen. The loop necessarily takes a small bite of tissue and it may become necessary to clear the loop before taking a second bite. Therefore this procedure may be very slow and cumbersome. Once again, the base should be biopsied and sent separately for staging purposes before it is ablated. A long standard resectoscope has also been used to resect a large volume tumor located in the distal ureter after previously dilating extensively the ureteral orifice [21].

Various forms of laser energy can be used to ablate the tumor base after its resection or to completely ablate/evaporate the tumor in its entirety. The ability of controlling the energy settings and the fact that the thermal effect on adjacent tissues declines with distance makes laser energy safe especially for the thin pelvic/ureteral wall. The risk for perforation is low thus decreasing the risk for stricture or tumor cell extravasation. Laser energy can be delivered with thin fibers that fit through flexible ureteroscopes without significantly altering irrigant flow or scope deflection. Minimal bleeding also aids in good visualization allowing for precise tumor ablation. Recently, laser energy with either holmium:yttrium-argon-garnet (Ho:YAG) or neodymium:yttrium-argon-garnet (Nd:YAG) sources have been popular.

Laser wavelength emission determines the degree of tissue absorption and thus depth of thermal injury, providing each type of laser with various advantages and disadvantages (Table 2). The Ho:YAG laser, operated usually at energy levels of 0.8–1.2J and at a frequency of 8–12Hz, has the ability to both coagulate and ablate tissue. This type of laser is particularly safe for use in the ureter because tissue penetration is less than 0.5mm, which allows for precise tumor ablation with minimal risk of full-thickness injury to the ureteral wall [22,23]. Its shallow penetration may, however, make its use cumbersome with larger tumors. Although rare if bleeding occurs, setting energy at lower levels or moving the fiber slightly away for the tissue will give a more diffuse effect that is more coagulative. This type of laser is particularly useful for ureteral lesions since it can ablate and remove a visually occlusive neoplasm. Alternatively, because of its ablative properties, the Ho:YAG laser has been used in conjunction with the Nd:YAG laser, in order to remove/ablate previously coagulated tissue [24,25].

The Nd:YAG laser works by coagulative necrosis with subsequent sloughing of the necrotic tumor [26]. The 5–6-mm penetration depth achieved with this type of laser allows coagulation of larger tumors but makes perforation of the

Table 2. Characteristics of holmium:yttrium-argon-garnet (Ho:YAG) and neodymium:yttrium-argon-garnet (Nd:YAG) laser energy sources

Ho:YAG	Nd:YAG
Minimal penetration (<0.5mm)	Deeper penetration (5–6mm)
Tumor destruction by ablation	Tumor destruction by coagulative necrosis
Precise cutting	Excellent hemostasis
Better for small ureteral tumors	Better for bulkier tumors

thin ureteral wall easier. The laser fiber should be always aimed parallel to the wall and coagulated tissue should be removed at regular intervals in order to evaluate the depth of tumor destruction. The laser fibers used are thin (1.8–2.1 F) and fit through both small-diameter rigid and flexible ureteroscopes. Care should be taken to avoid direct contact between the tissue and the tip of the fiber because the tip will then become charred. Settings most commonly used for the Nd:YAG laser are 15 W for 2 s for tumor ablation, and 5–10 W for 2 s for tissue coagulation.

When laser equipment is not available, electrocautery [27] via a small 2–3 F Bugbee electrode may be used to ablate ureteral tumors. In such cases water, sorbitol, or glycine as irrigation is necessary. Due to the risk of scarring and ureteral stenosis, the cutting current should be maintained at the lowest setting necessary for adequate tumor resection. Circumferential fulguration should be avoided for the same reason.

Irrespective of the technique used to remove a ureteral tumor, at the end of the procedure a double J stent is placed to prevent obstruction from edema or a blood clot. An open-ended ureteral stent may alternatively be used, especially if mitomycin instillation is planned postoperatively.

Complications

Complications associated with retrograde ureteroscopic treatment are uncommon and have decreased with improved instrumentation and refined technique [28].

Injury of the ureter may occur during dilatation of the ureteral orifice when larger diameter ureteroscopes are used. However, this rarely happens because dilatation is hardly ever needed with the new smaller ureteroscopes.

Ureteral perforation is also an uncommon complication with the proper technique. The gentle use of hydrophilic guide wires facilitates safe access to any part of the upper urinary tract. Maintaining clear vision and direct observation during biopsy or resection of the ureteral tumor helps decrease the risk for ureteral avulsion/perforation. Lasers should be used with appropriate power settings and ablation should always be performed with the laser fiber parallel to the ureteral wall to avoid the spread of thermal injury to the ureter. If a small perforation occurs the procedure may continue with minimal irrigation if a safety wire is present and good visualization is maintained. However, discontinuing the operation should be considered if tumor seeding is a concern. Extraluminal spillage or propagation of the neoplasm during endoscopic management of such tumors is a theoretical risk [29] although evidence of implantation throughout the ureter after ureteroscopy is lacking [30]. Most perforations are amenable to conservative treatment with a ureteral stent; however, if the tear is large percutaneous drainage may be considered.

The major long-term sequela of ureteroscopic management of upper tract urothelial tumors is postoperative ureteral stricture. This is frequently not secondary to injury during the ureteroscopic exploration but due to the to the type of energy used for tumor ablation. Fulguration must remain superficial, otherwise thermal damage with subsequent scarring and stricture of the ureteral wall may occur. Extensive tumors circumferentially located are at greater risk for postoperative stricture after therapy. Electrocautery causes the most extensive collateral thermal damage. Nd:YAG laser energy also creates a deep coagulative effect. However, in a study by Schmeller and Hofstetter [31] this form of energy, when used for conservative treatment of upper urinary tract tumors alone, caused less postoperative strictures compared with a combination of Nd:YAG laser and electroresection. We may expect even less ureteral damage with the use of a Ho:YAG laser because of its more limited tissue penetration. In fact no strictures were reported in a review of 22 patients with TCC of the ureter treated ureteroscopically with the Ho:YAG laser [32]. However, especially for high-grade tumors, one must keep in mind that strictures may be due to disease recurrence or inadequate resection. It is usually invading tumors that are inadequately removed, although this may be also happen with superficial tumors due to bad visualization from intraoperative bleeding. Strictured areas should be biopsied in order to determine the presence of malignancy. If residual disease is confirmed a radical nephroureterectomy must be considered. If benign, balloon dilatation or ureteroscopic incision may be performed, opening the ureteral lumen and facilitating subsequent ureteroscopic evaluations during follow-up.

Surveillance Protocol

Surveillance for recurrence is essential with endoscopic treatment of the upper urinary tract. Protocols may vary in detail but should be vigorous and lifelong. In our institution follow-up varies according to tumor grade and stage, but generally patients are evaluated every 3–6 months for a year, every 6 months for 4 years, and then yearly.

Follow-up visits always include history, physical examination, and urine cytology studies. Cystoscopy is also necessary due to the high incidence of recurrent bladder tumors in these patients, and should be performed along with the usual follow-up studies. Evaluation of the entire upper urinary tract can be done either by excretory urography or by retrograde ureteropyelography at 6-month intervals for the first 2 years and annually thereafter. Radiographic studies present with high rates of false-negative results [33,34] and therefore, many investigators prefer ureteroscopy since direct inspection has proven to be more sensitive in detecting tumor recurrence [35]. Because ureteroscopy is invasive it may alternatively be obtained yearly or when clinically indicated. Higher-grade lesions need to be followed more carefully and should include evaluation for metastatic disease with imaging of chest, abdomen, and pelvis. If the pathological results at any time reveal deeply invasive and/or high-grade carcinoma, or if there is a question of unresectable tumor, nephroureterectomy should be considered.

Adjuvant Instillation Therapy

Adjuvant therapy has no proven role but has been employed after ureteroscopic resection of urothelial tumors in an effort to decrease recurrences in these patients. Both immunotherapeutic and chemotherapeutic agents have been used.

Mitomycin C has been proven to be safe. Instillation is performed through an open-ended ureteral catheter [36]. The agent may also be administered by bladder instillation in the Trendelenberg position after double J insertion. However, the extent of urothelial exposure is variable and therefore the effectiveness has yet to be proven in larger series of patients. Alternatively, a nephrostomy tube may be placed and used for instillation of the therapeutic agent postoperatively.

The use of bacillus Calmette–Guerin (BCG) through retrograde ureteral catheters has been proposed [37], but not favored by everyone because of the potential to cause ureteral strictures. Negative urine cultures, cessation of hematuria, and confirmation of nonobstructive flow are necessary before administration of any agent is performed.

Results

Conservative management of upper urinary tract urothelial tumors requires lifelong vigilant follow-up for recurrence in the site of primary resection or elsewhere in the upper urinary tract. Recurrence in the bladder is seen in 30%–50% of patients [5,7] and requires cystoscopic surveillance as well.

Local control can be achieved with the ureteroscopic approach but long-term results vary from study to study due to the diversity of patient characteristics, follow-up patterns, and the small number of patients used in these cohorts (Table 3). Comparisons are affected by selection bias since some studies treat all patients, while others treat only those with a good prognosis. When comparing results with the gold standard nephroureterectomy, one must keep in mind the possibility of understaging of conservatively treated patients since pathologic staging is not available in all cases treated.

It is well established that tumor grade is the strongest prognostic indicator of recurrence and cancer-related deaths. Recurrence rates increased with increasing grade, and tumor progression was more frequent in grade III tumors [38]. Martinez-Pineiro et al. [39] proposed that the success rate of ureteroscopic therapy for grade I–II tumors is similar to bladder lesions of the same grade treated endoscopically, while no deep tumor invasion was seen in any of the patients with low-grade lesions. Tumor recurrence rates ranged from 27% for grade I tumors to 40% for grade II tumors. Similarly, Keeley et al. [25] reported a recurrence rate of 26% for grade I tumors and 44% for grade II tumors, which roughly correlated with previously established recurrence rates for open conservative surgery. Grade I tumors generally have a good prognosis and are the tumors preferred for ureteroscopic ablation. Newer long-term studies suggest

TABLE 3. Series of patients with upper tract urothelial tumors treated ureteroscopically

First author [Ref.]	Ureter	Resection modality	Recurrence of UUT TCC	Development of bladder tumor	Follow-up (months)	Open procedure required
Schmeller [31]	20	Nd	3	NA	5–22	4
Gaboardi [42]	18	Nd	8	NA	6–30	1
Elliott [38]	37	Nd/E	17	19	3–132	6
Martinez-Pineiro [39]	28	Nd/E	8	NA	2–119	3
Keeley [25]	41	Nd/Ho/E	8	15	3–116	8
Chen [43]	23	Nd/Ho/E	13	7	8–103	4
Elliot [44]	21	Nd/E	8	NA	12–73	4
Daneshmand [8]	26	Nd/Ho/E	23	7	2–106	9

Nd, Nd:YAG laser; Ho, Ho:YAG laser; E, electrocautery; UUT, upper urinary tract; TCC, transitional cell carcinoma.

more frequent recurrences than were previously reported. Daneshmand et al. [8] reported an average of 3.4 recurrences per patient with an average time of 7 months until first recurrence.

Although recurrences are expected in many patients after conservative management even for low-grade lesions, continued endoscopic management may successfully control the disease, with nephroureterectomy required only in up to 34.6% of patients, usually for high grade and progressive disease [8]. Recurrence does not depend on the initial tumor location site, since it was shown that tumors in the renal pelvis and ureter recur with similar frequency (31.2% and 33%, respectively) [40].

Ureteroscopic management is technically safe and complications are not frequent. The most frequent long-term sequela is ureteral stricture; however, local recurrence must always be ruled out before treating it as benign. There is no evidence of progression or spread of disease to other urothelial surfaces or metastatic sites with ureteroscopic management of such tumors. Kulp and Bagley [30] reported on 13 patients who underwent multiple ureteroscopic treatments followed by nephroureterectomy. They found no unusual propagation of transitional cell carcinoma in their specimens. Similarly, Hendin and colleagues [41] reported no increased risk of metastatic disease in a group of patients who underwent ureteroscopy before nephroureterectomy when compared with the group undergoing nephroureterectomy alone.

Tumor ablation modality is believed not to influence the success of conservative management despite the lack of large studies comparing success rates between various forms of energy sources. However, collateral thermal damage from different ablation sources may be responsible for the different stricture rates observed.

Conclusion

Ureteroscopic management of upper tract urothelial tumors is an established way of management for patients with solitary kidneys, bilateral disease, or compromised renal function. This kind of therapy is accepted for focal, low-grade superficial disease in patients with a normal contralateral kidney, provided that the patient is committed to lifelong endoscopic follow-up since recurrence is frequent even in patients with low-grade disease. However, salvage of renal units is obtained with adequate disease control. Patients with invasive or high grade disease are more likely to experience recurrence or progression, and often will eventually require radical nephroureterectomy. New ureteroscopic instrumentation of small diameter and grater flexibility allow for safe and efficient management of most small upper urinary tract tumors.

References

1. Silverberg E (1984) Cancer statistics. CA Cancer J Clin 34:7–23
2. McDonald MW, Zincke H (1987) Urothelial tumors of the upper urinary tract. In: deKernion JR, Paulson DF (eds) Genitourinary cancer management, 1st edn. Lea and Febiger, Philadelphia, pp 1–39
3. Murphy DM, Zincke H, Furlow WL (1980) Primary grade I transitional cell carcinoma of the renal pelvis and ureter. J Urol 123:629–633
4. Bennington JL, Beckwith JB (1975) Tumors of the kidney, renal pelvis, and ureter. In: Atlas of tumor pathology, 2nd series, fascicle 12. Armed Forces Institute of Pathology, Washington, DC
5. Oldbring J, Glifberg I, Mikulowski P, Hellsten S (1989) Carcinoma of the renal pelvis and ureter following bladder carcinoma: Frequency, risk factors, and clinicopathological findings. J Urol 141:1311–1313
6. Charbit L, Gendreau MC, Mee S, Cukier J (1991) Tumors of the upper urinary tract: 10 years experience. J Urol 146:1243–1246
7. Kang CH, Yu TJ, Hsieh HH, Yang JW, Shu K, Huang CC, Chiang PH, Shiue YL (2003) The development of bladder tumors and contralateral upper urinary tract tumors after primary transitional cell carcinoma of the upper urinary tract. Cancer 98:1620–1626
8. Daneshmand S, Quek ML, Huffman JL (2003) Endoscopic management of upper urinary tract transitional cell carcinoma: long-term experience. Cancer 98:55–60
9. Chesko SB, Gray GF, McCarron JP (1981) Urothelial neoplasia of the upper urinary tract. In: Sommers SC, Rosen PP (eds) Pathology annual, part 2. Appleton Century-Crofts, New York, pp 127–153
10. Heney NM, Nocks BN, Daly JJ, Blitzer PH, Parkhurst EC (1981) Prognostic factors in carcinoma of the ureter. J Urol 125:632–636
11. Badalament RA, Bennett WF, Bova JG, Kenworthy PR, Wise HA 2nd, Smith S, Perez J (1992) Computed tomography for detection and staging of transitional cell carcinoma of upper urinary tracts. Urology 40:71–75
12. Gerber GS, Lyon ES (1993) Endourological management of upper tract urothelial tumors. J Urol 150:2–7

13. Guarnizo E, Pavlovich CP, Seiba M, Carlson DL, Vaughan ED, Sosa RE (2000) Ureteroscopic biopsy of upper tract urothelial carcinoma: Improved diagnostic accuracy and histopathological considerations using a multi biopsy approach. J Urol 163: 52–55
14. Huffman, JL (2000) Management of upper transitional cell carcinomas. In: Volgelzang NJ, Scardino PT, Shipley WU, Coffey DS (eds) Genitourinary oncology, 2nd edn. Lippincott Williams and Wilkins, Philadelphia, pp 367–383
15. Murphy DP, Gill IS, Streem SB (2002) Evolving management of upper tract transitional cell carcinoma at a tertiary care center. J Endourol 16:483–487
16. Huang A, Low RK, White RD (1995) Nephrostomy tract tumor seeding following percutaneous manipulation of a urethral carcinoma. J Urol 153:1041–1042
17. Abdel-Razzak O, Bagley DH (1993) The 6.9F semi rigid ureteroscope in clinical use. Urology 41:45–48
18. Grasso M, Bagley A (1994) 7.5/8.2F actively deflectable, flexible ureteroscope: a new device for both diagnostic and therapeutic upper urinary tract endoscopy. Urology 43:435–441
19. Bian Y, Ehya H, Bagley DH (1995) Cytologic diagnosis of upper urinary tract neoplasms by ureteroscopic sampling. Acta Cytol 39:733–740
20. Tawfiek ER, Bibbo M, Bagley D (1997) Ureteroscopic biopsy: technique and specimen preparation. Urology 50:117–119
21. Jarrett TW, Lee CK, Pardalidis NP, Smith AD (1995) Extensive dilation of distal ureter for endoscopic treatment of large volume ureteral disease. J Urol 153:1214–1217
22. Bagley D, Erhard M (1995) Use of the holmium laser in the upper urinary tract. Tech Urol 1:25–30
23. Razvi HA, Chun SS, Denstedt JD, Sales JL (1995) Soft-tissue applications of the holmium: YAG laser in urology. J Endourol 9:387–390
24. Mills LW, Leniado ME, Patel A (2001) The role of endoscopy in the management of patients with upper urinary transitional cell carcinoma. BJU Int 87:150–162
25. Keeley FX, Bibbo M, Bagley DH (1997) Ureteroscopic treatment and surveillance of upper tract transitional cell carcinoma. J Urol 157:1560–1565
26. Kaufman RP, Carson CC (1993) Ureteroscopic management of transitional cell carcinoma of the ureter using the Neodymium:YAG laser. Lasers Surg Med 13:625–628
27. Huffman JL, Bagley DH, Lyon ES, Morse MJ, Herr HW, Whitmore WF Jr (1985) Endoscopic diagnosis and treatment of upper tract urothelial tumors. Cancer 55:1422–1428
28. Grasso M, Bagley D (1997) Small diameter actively deflectable, flexible ureteropyeloscopy. J Urol 157:28–32
29. Lim DJ, Shattuck MO, Cock WA (1993) Pyelovenous lymphatic migration of transitional cell carcinoma following flexible ureterorenoscopy. J Urol 149:109–111
30. Kulp DA, Bagley DH (1994) Does flexible ureteropyeloscopy promote local recurrence of transitional cell carcinoma? J Endourol 8:111–113
31. Schmeller NT, Hofstetter AG (1989) Laser treatment of ureteral tumors. J Urol 141:1298–1301
32. Chen GL, Bagley DH (2001) Ureteroscopic surgery for upper tract transitional cell carcinoma: complications and management. J Endourol 15:399–404
33. Grossman HB, Schwartz SL, Konnak JW (1992) Ureteroscopic treatment of urothelial carcinoma of the ureter and renal pelvis. J Urol 148:275–277

34. Bagley DH (1993) Ureteroscopic treatment of ureteral and renal pelvic tumors: extended follow-up. J Urol 149:492A
35. Richie JP (1988) Carcinoma of the renal pelvis and ureter. In: Skinner DG, Lieskovsky G (eds) Diagnosis and management of genitourinary cancer. Saunders, Philadelphia, pp 323–336
36. Eastham JA, Huffman JL (1993) Technique of Mitomycin C instillation in the treatment of upper urinary tract urothelial tumors. J Urol 150:324–325
37. Sharpe JR, Duffy G, Chin JL (1993) Intrarenal bacillus Calmette-Guerin therapy for upper urinary tract carcinoma in situ. J Urol 149:457–460
38. Elliott DS, Blute ML, Patterson DE, Bergstralh EJ, Segura JW (1996) Long term follow-up of endoscopically treated upper urinary tract transitional cell carcinoma. Urology 47:819–825
39. Martinez-Pineiro JA, Matres Garcia MJ, Martinez Pineiro L (1996) Endourological treatment of upper tract urothelial carcinomas: Analysis of a series of 59 tumors. J Urol 156:377–385
40. Tawfiek ER, Bagley DH (1997) Upper tract transitional cell carcinoma. Urology 50:321–329
41. Hendin BN, Streem SB, Levin HS, Klein EA, Novick AC. Impact of diagnostic ureteroscopy on long-term survival in patients with upper tract transitional cell carcinoma. J Urol 1999;161:783–785
42. Gaboardi F, Bozzola A, Dotti E, Galli L (1994) Conservative treatment of upper urinary tract tumors with Nd:YAG laser. J Endourol 8:37–41
43. Chen GL, Bagley DH (2000) Ureteroscopic management of upper tract transitional cell carcinoma in patients with normal contralateral kidneys. J Urol 164:1173–1176
44. Elliott DS, Segura JW, Lightner D, Patterson DE, Blute ML (2001) Is nephroureterectomy necessary in all cases of upper tract transitional cell carcinoma? Long term results of conservative endourologic management of upper tract transitional cell carcinoma in individuals with a normal contralateral kidney. Urology 58:174–178

Laparoscopic Nephroureterectomy for Upper Urinary Tract Transitional Cell Carcinoma: A Review of the Current Literature

Jens J. Rassweiler, Michael Schulze, Dogu Teber, Svetozar Subotic, and Thomas Frede

Summary. In 1991, laparoscopic nephroureterectomy was been introduced as a treatment option for upper tract transitional cell carcinoma. Based on personal long-term experience and the review of the current literature, we analyzed the actual results of this technique in comparison to open surgery. We reviewed the charts and followed up 23 patients who underwent laparoscopic nephroureterectomy at the Klinikum Heilbronn between December 1994 and December 2003, and 21 patients who underwent open nephroureterectomy during the same period. Demographic, perioperative, and follow-up data were compared. Additionally, we performed a MEDLINE/PUBMED search and reviewed the literature on laparoscopic and open nephroureterectomy between 1991 and 2004 (n = 1365 patients). The analysis of the literature including the Heilbronn experience revealed a slightly longer operating time (276.6 vs 220.1 min), and significantly lower blood loss (240.9 vs 462.9 ml) in the laparoscopic series. No differences of minor (12.9% vs 14.1%) or major complication rates (5.6% vs 8.3%) were observed. All nine comparative studies revealed a significant dose reduction of the morphine equivalents after laparoscopy. In all ten comparative series the hospital stay was shorter after laparoscopy, but only in six series was the difference statistically significant. The frequency of bladder recurrence (24.0% vs 24.7%), local recurrence (4.4% vs 6.3%), and distant metastases (15.5% vs 15.2%) did not differ significantly in both groups. The actual disease-free 2-year survival rates (75.2% vs 76.2%) were similar. The 5-year survival rates averaged 81.2% in the three laparoscopic (n = 113 patients) and 61% in the ten open series (n = 681 patients). Six port site metastases were reported in 377 (1.6%) analyzed patients occurring 3–12 months following laparoscopy. Open radical nephroureterectomy still represents the gold standard for the management of upper tract transitional cell carcinoma; however, laparoscopic radical nephroureterectomy offers the advantages of minimally invasive surgery without

Department of Urology, University of Heidelberg, SLK Kliniken Heilbronn, Am Gesundbrunnen 20, D-74078 Heilbronn, Germany

deterioration in the oncological outcome. In cases of advanced tumors (pT3, N+), open surgery is still recommended.

Keywords. Carcinoma, Transitional cell carcinoma, Kidney, Nephroureterectomy, Laparoscopic surgical procedure, Port site metastasis

Introduction

Conventional open complete nephroureterectomy with excision of the ipsilateral orifice and a bladder cuff has been the accepted standard operative therapy for most patients with upper tract transitional cell carcinoma [1–8]. This approach requires one or two long incisions associated with respective morbidity. Therefore, based on the first report of McDonald et al. in 1952 [9], several authors tried to minimize the access trauma by use of an endoscopic transurethral detachment technique of the distal ureter [10–17].

In 1991, Clayman and colleagues first described the technique of laparoscopic nephroureterectomy [18,19], which was soon replicated by various authors worldwide [20–23]. However, particularly due to major concerns about the oncological outcome, there was only a limited spread of the technique in the following years. With increasing acceptance of laparoscopic radical nephrectomy for renal cell cancer, however, several centers have recently reported their initial experiences [24–29]. Additionally, some authors compared their data with the results of contemporary patients treated by open nephroureterectomy [30–47] and one international multicenter study even presented short-term oncological data [48].

Based on a point–counterpoint discussion at the recent EAU Congress in Vienna, we wish to present an overview of the current data in the literature including an update of our own personal experience. In this analysis special emphasis is placed on the criteria of evidence-based medicine, thus representing an update of the recently published EAU guidelines of laparoscopy [49].

Materials and Methods

In this chapter we analyze the current literature as well as our own patients treated by open or laparoscopic nephroureterectomy, focusing on technical aspects (i.e., type of access, method of ureterectomy), perioperative data (i.e., operating time, complications, pain), and oncological parameters (local recurrence, bladder tumor, distant metastasis, survival).

Heilbronn Experience

We reviewed the charts and followed up 23 patients (mean age 62.2 years, range 43–80) who underwent laparoscopic retroperitoneal nephroureterectomy between December 1994 and December 2003 and 21 patients (mean age 70.5 years, range 57–80) who underwent open nephroureterectomy during the same period at the Klinikum Heilbronn. Male-to-female ratio, distribution of side, and site of the upper tract transitional cell carcinoma were similar in both groups (Table 1a). The same surgeons performed both procedures. Demographic, perioperative, and follow-up data were compared.

The technique of retroperitoneoscopic radical nephrectomy has been previously described in detail [50–52]. Open radical nephrectomy was performed via a supracostal flank incision above the 11th rib. Ureterectomy was performed by two different techniques. In one patient of the laparoscopic and three of the open group, a completely endoscopic ureterectomy was realized by transurethral circumcision of the orifice prior to retroperitoneoscopy using a Turner–Warwick hook after stenting the ureter. In this technique the intramural part of the ureter is completely isolated until it retracts into the extraperitoneal space. Now the patient is positioned as for radical nephrectomy, and the ureter is primarily dis-

TABLE 1a. Laparoscopic vs open retroperitoneal nephroureterectomy—Heilbronn experience: patient data

Criteria	Retroperitoneal nephroureterectomy	
	Laparoscopic	Open
Total number	23	21
Age (range)	62.2 (43–80)	70.5 (57–80)
Male/female	13/9	15/6
Left/right	12/11	14/7
Kidney/ureter	14/9	17/4
Median tumor size (cm)	2.75 (1–14)	4.0 (2–8)
Tumor staging		
pTa	12	3
pT1	4	5
pT2	3	3
pT3	4	8
pT4	—	2
G1	1	—
G2	12	8
G3	10	13
Access		
Transperitoneal	2	2
Retroperitoneal	20	18
Technique of ureterectomy		
Open incision	21	16
Transurethral circumcison	1	3
No ureterectomy	1	1
Specimen retrieval		
Morcellation	0	0
By incision	23	20

sected and clipped to prevent tumor cell spillage along the stent. At this stage radical nephrectomy is accomplished, the ureter is antegradely dissected towards the bladder, and is thereafter extracted en bloc. In 21 laparoscopic and 16 open patients, we preferred the retrieval of the entire kidney specimen via a suprainguinal incision to avoid morcellation. This access was then used for open dissection of the distal ureter including a bladder cuff. One patient in each group had no ureterectomy, because transitional cell carcinoma was detected surprisingly instead of a renal cell carcinoma.

Analysis of the Literature

We conducted an extensive MEDLINE/PUBMED search of laparoscopic and open nephroureterectomy from 1991 through 2004. Articles published earlier than 1991 have been included selectively (Table 2). Apart from reasonable exceptions, only full-length, English-language articles were considered for this review ($n = 85$). In cases of multiple reports from respective centers, only the last paper has been summarized in the tables. The overall mean values have been calculated on the basis of the mean values of each series and the number of patients having adequate data regarding the specific topic (e.g., operating time, bladder recurrence rate). Two-year survival rates of long-term studies were calculated according to Kaplan–Meier curves.

Statistical Analysis

All data of our patients were recorded prospectively in a database (Excel, Microsoft). The statistical analysis was performed using a commercial software package (SPSS, Microsoft). The differences between the stratified groups of our own results as well as from the literature research were analyzed using the chi-square test. Any P-value of less than 0.05 was considered as statistically significant.

Results

Heilbronn Experience

The tumor size did not differ significantly in both groups; however, significantly less pTa-tumors were treated by open surgery (Table 1a). Access as well as technique of ureterectomy and specimen retrieval was similar in both groups. The mean operating time of the laparoscopic group was slightly longer (200 vs 188 min) and the median blood loss slightly less (450 vs 600 ml), but the differences were not statistically significant. There were two conversions to open surgery in the laparoscopic group, both because of intraoperative hemorrhage. The overall complication rate was lower in the laparoscopic group (17.4% vs 23.8%), but again the difference was not statistically significant. One patient died

60 days after a left laparoscopic radical nephroureterectomy due to recurrent bleeding from the duodenal-pancreatic artery despite multiple open reinterventions. Overall reintervention rate (8.7% vs 4.8%) did not differ in both groups. One laparoscopic patient who required conversion to open surgery developed a hernia at the incision site (Table 1b). The median dosage of morphine equivalent (i.e., piritramide) was significantly lower in the laparoscopic group (18 vs 33 mg). The median hospital stay was shorter after laparoscopy (10 vs 13 days), but the difference was not statistically significant.

The mean observation time was almost identical in both groups (50 vs 54 months). In this period of time, 34.8% of the laparoscopic patients experienced a bladder tumor compared with 14.4% after open surgery ($P > 0.05$) (Fig. 1). On the other hand, 17.4% developed distant metastases after laparoscopic and 28.5% after open surgery; however, this difference was not statistically significant.

Overall 5-year disease-free survival was 81% after laparoscopic and 63% after open surgery (Fig. 2). The differences for pTa/T1-tumors (85% vs 100%) as well as for pT2/3 stages (75% vs 45%) were not statistically significant (Table 1c).

Analysis of the Literature

The results of 1365 patients, 402 (29.8%) of whom were part of a comparative study, were evaluated. The data of 116 patients were collected in a single multicenter study (Table 2).

TABLE 1b. Laparoscopic vs open retroperitoneal nephroureterectomy—Heilbronn experience: perioperative data

Criteria	Retroperitoneal nephroureterectomy	
	Laparoscopic	Open
Operating time (min)	200 (125–333)	188 (140–349)
Median blood loss (ml)	450 (200–3500)	600 (500–1600)
Conversion to open surgery (%)	2 (8.7%)s	—
Complications	4 (17.4)%	5 (23.8)%
Bleeding	3	—
Pleura lesion	—	2
Wound healing	1	—
Cerebral bleeding	—	1
Hernia	—	2
Mortality (after 60 days)	1	—
Reintervention	2 (8.7)	1 (4.8%)
Early	1	1
Late	2[a]	—
Median analgesics (morphine-equivalent) (mg)	18 (5–67)	33 (20–128)
Median hospital stay (days)	10 (7–60)	13 (7–34)

[a] Hernia after conversion to open surgery.

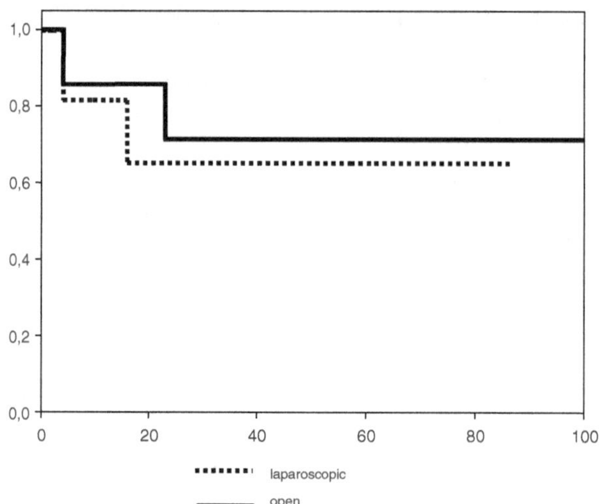

Fig. 1. Bladder recurrences in pTa or pT1-Tumors following laparoscopic/open radical nephroureterectomy (postoperative follow-up in months)

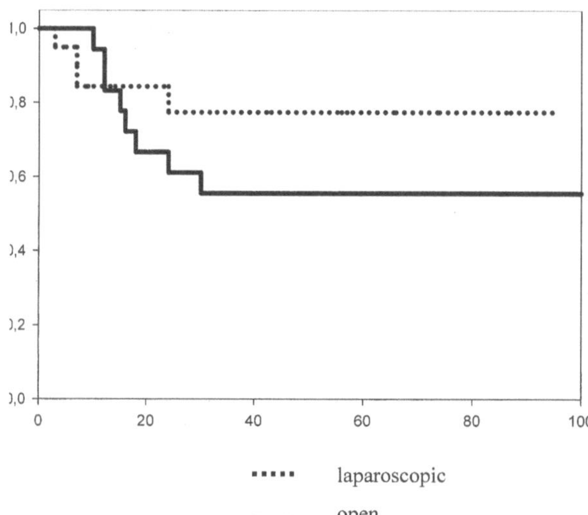

Fig. 2. Overall survival rates following laparoscopic/open radical nephroureterectomy (postoperative follow-up in months)

Table 1c. Laparoscopic vs open retroperitoneal nephroureterectomy—Heilbronn experience: follow-up data

Criteria	Retroperitoneal nephroureterectomy	
	Laparoscopic	Open
Total no.	23	21
Observation time (months)	50 (2–110)	54 (2–102)
Bladder recurrence (%)	8 (34.8)	3 (14.4)
Local recurrence (%)	0	1 (4.8)
Distant metastases	4 (17.4)	6 (28.5%)
Dead of disease	4	7
Dead of other causes	2	2
Overall survival	74%	57%
Disease-free survival (5 years)		
Overall	81%	63%
pTa/T1	85%	100%
pT2/T3	75%	45%

TABLE 2. Management of upper tract transitional cell carcinoma: distribution of 1186 patients being reviewed in the current literature

Procedure	Overall no. pts	Comparative study (no. of studies)	Multicenter studies (no. of studies)
Open nephroureterectomy	969	200 (8)	None
Laparoscopic nephroureterectomy	377	202 (8)	116 (1)
Total	1365	402	116

Operative Data (Tables 3a and b)

Concerning the access (i.e. trans-, retroperitoneal), there is no preference in the literature. Some groups tried a hand-assisted technique, which seems reasonable, because the preferred intact removal of the specimen requires an incision of at least 6–8 cm. This incision can also be used for ureterectomy with open bladder cuff, which has been applied by 10 of the 17 (58.8%) groups, whereas in the multicenter trial it was used in only 27% (Table 4). Other techniques include laparoscopic dissection of the distal ureter with extravesical stapling of the bladder wall (i.e., with an Endo-GIA stapler), the transurethral circumcision of the orifice and antegrade stripping (i.e., "pluck-off technique"), and the transvesical endoscopic detachment of the ureter (Cleveland technique). Interestingly, the minimally invasive techniques of ureterectomy, which could all be applied by open surgery, did not play a significant role in the reported cases of open surgery (i.e., comparative studies; Table 3).

The mean operating time ranged from 165 and 462 (mean 276.6) min in the laparoscopic ($n = 324$ patients) and from 165 to 280 (mean 220.1) min in the open series ($n = 257$ patients). Only three of ten comparative studies showed significantly longer operating times for laparoscopy; all these came from the United States. The blood loss ranged between 140 and 462 (mean 240.9) ml in the laparoscopic ($n = 268$ patients) and from 240 to 696 (mean 462.9) ml in the open series ($n = 220$ patients). All nine comparative studies demonstrated significantly less blood loss after laparoscopy.

Postoperative Course (Table 3c)

The rate of minor complications ranged between 0% and 40% (mean 12.9%) in the laparoscopic ($n = 312$ patients) and from 0% to 45% (mean 14.1%) in the open series ($n = 206$ patients). Major complications occurred in 0%–19% (mean 5.6%) in the laparoscopic and 0%–29% (mean 8.3%) in the open series. All nine comparative studies revealed a significant dose reduction of the morphine-equivalents after laparoscopy. According to the different healthcare systems (i.e., Europe, United States), the absolute length of hospital stay differed significantly within each series (2.3–13.0 vs 4.6–13.3 days). In all ten comparative series the hospital stay was shorter after laparoscopy, but only in six series was the difference statistically significant.

Table 3a. Laparoscopic vs open radical nephroureterectomy operative data: laparoscopic radical nephroureterectomy

First author [Ref.] Year	*n*	Technique of nephrectomy	Technique of ureterectomy	Operating time (min)	Blood loss (ml)
Chung [25] 1996	7	Retroperitoneal	Open bladder	275	n.a.
Barrett [26] 1998	22	Transperitoneal	Open Bladder	200	n.a.
Shalhav [30] 2000	25	Transperitoneal	Extravesical stapling	462	199[a]
McNeill [31] 2000	25	Transperitoneal	Transurethral resection	165	n.a.[a]
Gill [32] 2000	42	Retroperitoneal	Transvesical detachment	269	242[a]
Stifelman [33] 2001	11	Transperiton. hand-assisted	Transvesical detachment	291	147[a]
Seifman [34] 2001	16	Transperiton. hand-assisted	Transurethral resection/open bladder cuff	320	288[a]
Jarrett [35] 2001	25	Transperitoneal	Extravesical stapling/open bladder cuff	329	440
Chen [36] 2001	7	Transperiton. hand-assisted	Open bladder cuff	n.a.	140[a]
Uozumi [37] 2002	10	Retroperiton hand-assisted	Open bladder cuff	456	462
Landman [38] 2002	16	Transperiton. hand-assisted	Extravesical stapling + TUR	294	201
Matsui [39] 2002	17	Retroperitoneal	Open bladder cuff	287	151[a]
Goel [40] 2002	9	Retroperitoneal	Open bladder cuff	189	n.a.
Kawauchi [42] 2003	34	Retroperitoneal	Open bladder cuff/transurethral resection	233	236[a]
Yoshino [44] 2003	23	Retroperitoneal	Extravesical stapling	330	304
Klingler [45] 2003	19	Trans-/retroperitoneal[c]	Open bladder cuff	198	282[a]
Rassweiler 2004[b]	23	Retroperitoneal	Open bladder cuff	200	450[a]

n.a., not available.

[a] Comparative study.

[b] Present study.

[c] In 14/19 with ipsilateral lymphadenectomy.

TABLE 3b. Laparoscopic vs open radical nephroureterectomy operative data: open radical nephroureterectomy

First author [Ref.] Year	*n*	Technique of nephrectomy	Technique of ureterectomy	Operating time (min)	Blood loss (ml)
Angulo [15] 1998	19	Retroperitoneal	Transurethral	168	240
Angulo [15] 1998	15	Retroperitoneal	Open bladder cuff	204	392
Shalhav [30] 2000	17	Retroperitoneal	Open bladder cuff	234	441[a]
McNeill [31] 2000	42	Retroperitoneal	Open bladder cuff	165	n.a.[a]
Gill [32] 2000	35	Trans-/ retroperitoneal	Open bladder cuff	280	696[a]
Stifelman [33] 2001	11	Retroperitoneal	Open bladder cuff	232	311[a]
Seifman [34] 2001	11	Retroperitoneal	Open bladder cuff	199	345[a]
Chen [36] 2001	15	Retroperitoneal	Open bladder cuff	222	455[a]
Matsui [39] 2002	17	Retroperitoneal	Open bladder cuff	240	300[a]
Goel [40] 2002	5	Retroperitoneal	Open bladder cuff	184	n.a.[a]
Kawauchi [42] 2003	34	Retro-/ transperitoneal	Open bladder cuff/ transurethral resection	236	427[a]
Klingler [45] 2003	15	Transperitoneal	Open bladder cuff	220	532[a]
Rassweiler 2004[b]	21	Retroperitoneal	Open bladder cuff	188	600[a]

[a] Comparative study.
[b] Present study.

Oncological Follow-Up (Table 5)

It has to be emphasized that apart from the present study only two further laparoscopic studies provide an observation time of at least 5 years. Most papers report 2-year results maximally. During this period of time, bladder recurrence occurred in 9%–48% (mean 24.0%) in the laparoscopic (n = 342 patients) and in 13.3%–53.8% (mean 24.7%) in the open series (n = 705 patients). Local recurrence was documented as between 0% and 15.3% (mean 4.4%) in the laparoscopic (n = 250 patients) and between 0% and 15.4% (mean 6.3%) in the open series (n = 607 patients). Distant metastases were found in the range of 6%–28% (mean 15.5%) in the laparoscopic (n = 349 patients) and from 0% to 29.2% (mean 15.2%) in the open series (n = 580 patients). Actual disease-free 2-year survival ranged between 69% and 94.7% (mean 75.2%) in the laparoscopic series (n = 285 patients) and between 69% and 93.7% (mean 76.2%) in the open series (n = 595 patients).

The 5-year survival rates range from 56% to 91% (mean 81.2%) in the three laparoscopic series (n = 113 patients) and from 49% to 83% (mean 61%) in the ten open series (n = 681 patients).

TABLE 3c. Laparoscopic vs open radical nephroureterectomy: postoperative course

First author [Ref.] Year	*n*	Complications (%)		Analgesics (mg)	Hospital stay (days)
		Minor	Major		
Laparoscopic radical nephroureterectomy					
Chung [25] 1996	7	14	0	12	9.0
Barrett [26] 1998	22	14	5	n.a.	8.5
Shalhav [30] 2000	25	40	8	37	6.1[a]
McNeill [31] 2000	25	12	4	n.a.	7.8[a]
Gill [32] 2000	42	7	5	26	2.3[a]
Stifelman [33] 2001	16	0	0	45	4.6[a]
Seifman [34] 2001	16	19	19	48	3.9[a]
Jarrett [35] 2001	25	24	12	n.a.	4.0
Chen [36] 2001	7	n.a.	n.a.	38	7.3[a]
Uozumi [37] 2002	10	30	10	n.a.	n.a.
Landman [38] 2002	16	25	6	33	4.5
Goel [40] 2002	9	0	0	275	5.1[a]
Kawauchi [42] 2003	34	6	6	2.1[d]	13.0[a]
Yoshino [44] 2003	23	0	0	60	n.a.
Klingler [45] 2003	19	0	0	190	8.1[a]
Rassweiler 2004[b]	23	9	9	18	10.0[a]
Open radical nephroureterectomy					
Angulo [15] 1998	19	5	0	n.a.	4.6
Angulo [15] 1998	15	7	7	n.a.	7.2
Shalhav [30] 2000	17	29	29	144	12.0[a]
McNeill [31] 2000	42	12	5	n.a.	10.7[a]
Gill [32] 2000	35	5	5	228	6.6[a]
Stifelman [33] 2001	11	10	0	44[c]	6.1[a]
Seifman [34] 2001	11	45	27	81	5.1[a]
Chen [36] 2001	15	n.a.	n.a.	70	9.1[a]
Goel [40] 2002	5	0	0	650	9.2[a]
Kawauchi [42] 2003	34	12	0	4.1[d]	21.1[a]
Klingler [45] 2003	15	13	13	590	13.3[a]
Rassweiler 2004[b]	21	14	10	33	13.0[a]

[a] Comparative study.
[b] Present study.
[c] Plus epidural analgesia.
[d] Frequency of parenteral analgesia.

TABLE 4. Laparoscopic radical nephroureterectomy: technique of ureterectomy (from El Fettouh et al. [48], International multicenter study, $n = 116$)

Technique	n (%)
Transvesical laparoscopic detachment and ligation technique	40 (34%)
Transurethral circumcision/resection of orifice with antegrade stripping	12 (10%)
Ureteral deroofing with extravesical stapling	31 (26%)
Open bladder cuff	33 (27%)

TABLE 5. Laparoscopic vs open radical nephroureterectomy: oncological results

First author [Ref.] Year	*n*	Bladder recurrence (%)	Local recurrence (%)	Distant metastasis	Survival at	
					2 years	5 years
Laparoscopic radical nephroureterectomy						
Barrett [26] 1998	22	22.7	4.5[b]	13.6	91	n.a.
Shalhav [30] 2000	13	23	15.3	15.3	77	n.a.[a]
Cicco [68] 2000	7	n.a.	14.1	14.1	69	n.a.
McNeill [31] 2000	25	28	8	28.0	74	56[a]
Jarrett [35] 2001	25	48	8	16.0	86	n.a.
El Fettouh [48] 2002	116	24	1.7	9.4	87	n.a.[c]
Kawauchi [42] 2003	34	9	0	6	n.a.	n.a.
Hattori [46] 2003	65	22	n.a.	28.0	n.a.	91[a]
Klingler [45] 2003	19	10.5	5.3	10.5	94.7	n.a.
Rassweiler 2004[d]	23	34.8	0	17.4	89	81[a]
Open radical nephroureterectomy						
Corrado [3] 1991	124	n.a.	n.a.	n.a.	81	67
Charbit [4] 1991	92	25.2	8.7	19.5	76	67[e]
Komatsu [65] 1991	36	36	11.1	11.1	n.a.	74[e]
Jurincic-Winkler [5] 1993	54	18.5	n.a.	n.a.	71	62
Hall [7] 1998	194	13.5	3.9	5.9	n.a.	49
Angulo [15] 1998	15	20	0	13.3	80	n.a.
Miyake [66] 1998	35	n.a.	n.a.	29.2[f]	78	58[e]
Miyake [66] 1998	37	n.a.	n.a.	29.2[f]	72	50
Shalhav [30] 2000	13	53.8	0	23	69	n.a.[a]
McNeill [31] 2000	42	42	15.4	18	68	64[a]
Salvador-Bayarri [17] 2002	145	37	0	n.a	84.2	n.a.
Kawauchi [42] 2003	34	38	0	9	n.a.	n.a.[a]
Hattori [46] 2003	44	45	n.a.	25	n.a.	83[a]
Klingler [45] 2003	15	13.3	6.6	6.6	93.7	n.a.[a]
Rassweiler 2004[d]	21	14.4	4.8	28.5	83	63[a]

[a] Comparative study.
[b] One port site metastasis.
[c] Multicenter study.
[d] Present study.
[e] Lymphadenectomy in all or most cases.
[f] Of all 72 cases.

Port Site Metastases (Table 6)

In 6 of the total of 377 (1.6%) patients analyzed in the review of the literature, port site metastases were reported to occur after 3–12 months. Interestingly, in all cases no organ bag ($n = 5$) was used or the bag was torn during retrieval of the specimen ($n = 1$). In two cases, the pathological finding was unexpected [transitional cell carcinoma (TCC) instead of tuberculosis, squamous cell carcinoma instead of TCC], and in one case there was conversion to open surgery due to intraoperative bleeding. Four patients experienced short-term metastatic progression of the tumor.

TABLE 6. Laparoscopic radical nephroureterectomy: port site metastases

First author [Ref.] Year	Stage	Grade	Interval	Specimen removal	Comments
Barrett [26] 1998	pT1	2	n.a.	Intact via incision, no bag	Metastatic disease (TCC) also, chemotherapy (alive 40 months)
Ahmed [69] 1998	pT2	3	8 months	Intact via incision, no bag	Also local recurrence and hepatic metastases (TCC), palliative chemotherapy
Otani [70] 1999	pT3	3	3 months	Intact via incision, bag torn	Pre- and intraoperatively TCC not known (tuberculous atrophic kidney)
Ong [71] 2003	pT1	3	12 months	Intact via incision, EndoCatch bag	Wide excision of masses (TCC)
Matsui [72] 2004	pT3	3	6 months	Intact via incision, no bag	Squamous cell carcinoma, 2 courses of adjuvant chemotherapy
Naderi [73] 2004	pT2	3	3 months	Intact via open surgery, no bag	Conversion to open surgery due to bleeding from renal vein, also metastasis at subcostal incision, chemotherapy only with partial remission

TCC, transitional cell carcinoma.

Discussion

The advantages of laparoscopic nephrectomy for benign disease have been well proven in several comparative studies revealing a significant reduction of post-operative morbidity [53,54]. However, in cases with oncological indications, such advantages have to be balanced against possible risks such as port site metastases or local recurrences [55,56]. Moreover, long-term follow-up is necessary to evaluate the oncological outcome in comparison to open and endourological techniques [57,58]. More than 10 years after the first description of a laparoscopic nephroureterectomy, it seems appropriate to analyze the current status of this technique in the management of upper tract TCC.

Technical Aspects

As in open surgery, there are several technical modifications of the procedure with respect to nephrectomy as well as regards the method of ureterectomy. Laparoscopic nephroureterectomy can be performed via a transperitoneal or a retroperitoneal access, in a pure laparoscopic or hand-assisted technique. Centers with long-term experience prefer the laparoscopic technique, because the hand-assisted surgery represents a compromise between the open and the laparoscopic approach. The advocates of the hand-assisted technique emphasize the shorter learning curve of the procedure as well as the ability of palpation. Additionally, since intact specimen retrieval is preferred, a larger skin incision is required. Definitively, the current data do not show any significant difference (i.e., with respect to postoperative morbidity) when comparing both techniques [59].

Additionally, the technique of ureterectomy has not been standardized yet, and will not be in the near future. Some authors feel that there might be a dilemma [60]; however, as nicely reviewed for open surgery by Laguna and de la Rosette [16], the outcome of all different techniques (Table 4) is quite similar. According to some anecdotal case reports [16,60–64], there might be a slightly higher risk of local progression when the transurethral pluck-off technique is used; however, the outcome analysis of all laparoscopic cases did not show any significant impact of the technique of ureterectomy (Table 5). Following extravesical dissection of a bladder cuff with use of endoscopic stapling devices, titanium staple lines can be seen endoscopically with the potential risk of stone formation [65]. According to our personal experience, there is a trend towards use of the open bladder cuff using the suprainguinal incision simultaneously for intact retrieval of the specimen. Moreover, there are no contraindications such as ureteral tumors or periureteral fibrosis due to previous surgery, irradiation, or inflammatory pelvic diseases [16,60]. Evidently, in contrast to open surgery (i.e., significant reduction of morbidity, shorter operating time) for the laparoscopic approach, the endoscopic techniques of ureterectomy play only a minor role.

Indications and Contraindications

Although comparable long-term results after endourological treatment (i.e., ureteroscopy, percutaneous tumor resection) for upper tract tumors have been reported [58] for selective series (i.e., bilateral tumors, single kidneys), there is still a consensus that upper tract transitional cell carcinoma requires radical nephroureterectomy. As in the Heilbronn series (Table 1), predominantly noninvasive tumors (pTa/pT1) have been treated laparoscopically; however, all series also include pT2 and pT3 stages. Since there is only limited experience with advanced stages (i.e., lymph node involvement), such cases still represent an indication for open surgery.

The role of lymph node dissection has not yet been defined, neither for open nor for laparoscopic radical nephroureterectomy. There are only two reports following open surgery and a single study after laparoscopy focusing on this issue [45,66,67]. Myake et al. [66] did not find any significant difference in 5-year survival rates of patients with and without ipsilateral lymph node dissection (Table 5). The curative effect of lymph node dissection is limited to pN1 stages, and the overall efficacy of adjuvant polychemotherapy for transitional cell cancer is still under debate. Moreover, tumor cell invasion of lymphatic vessels seem to correlate with the presence of lymph node metastases and represent an unfavorable prognostic factor [67]. Based on this, the indication for any kind of adjuvant chemotherapy should be based on lymphovascular tumor invasion in the specimen rather than on the histopathological results of a lymph node dissection.

Perioperative Outcome

The operative time was longer in the laparoscopic series (277 vs 200 min). However, this was mainly due to the early American studies. In the recently published European series (including the Heilbronn experience) the duration of laparoscopy did not differ significantly from open surgery. On the other hand, the blood loss was less (241 vs 463 ml), the dosage of analgesics lower, and the hospital stay shorter after laparoscopic nephroureterectomy (Table 3). No statistical significance was found with respect to overall complication rates (18% vs 21%). This indicates that laparoscopic radical nephroureterectomy has been established worldwide at centers of expertise as a safe and reproducible, minimally invasive technique. Operating time is still longer, but one may expect only marginal differences between both approaches in the near future. The similar complication rates reflect the fact that the learning curve of laparoscopic nephroureterectomy has plateaued—at least at the centers of expertise.

Oncological Outcome

It has to be emphasized that only three laparoscopic studies provide an observation time of at least 5 years, and this includes a total of 113 patients. Most of the other reports provide only a 2-year follow-up. Nevertheless, there were no statistically significant differences concerning all relevant results, such as bladder recurrences (24% vs 25%), local recurrence rate (4% vs 6%), and the occurrence of distant metastases (15.5% vs 15.1%) when comparing laparoscopic with open series. Moreover, the 2-year survival rates were almost identical (75% vs 76%). The 5-year survival rates of the laparoscopic series were slightly better (81% vs 61%); however, this might be attributable to a different case selection with more invasive tumors in the open series. In all three comparative long-term series (Edinburgh, Nagoya, Heilbronn) no significant differences were documented (Table 5). This is in accordance with the results of radical laparoscopic surgery for renal cell carcinoma [68].

Besides the overall oncological outcome, there is a general concern about technically specific risks, such as port site metastases following laparoscopy or local recurrences after transurethral detachment of the orifice [16,55,56,69]. In the meantime, six cases of port site metastases have been reported (Table 6), which may represent an incidence of 1.6% [26,70–74]. In contrast to other urological tumors (i.e., prostate carcinoma), the TCC is relatively aggressive. In the case of direct contact with the tumor, i.e., as reported by Bangma et al. [74] during laparoscopic pelvic lymph node dissection or Andersen and Steven [75] following laparoscopic biopsy of a bladder tumor, there is an increased risk of tumor cell spillage. In accordance to this, there are several reports of tract recurrences following intraoperative pyeloscopy [76], percutaneous renal surgery [77–79] or even biopsy [80].

However, if the patient is treated adequately after the procedure (i.e., by adjuvant chemotherapy), the risk of port site metastasis can be reduced. In the Heilbronn series of open nephroureterectomy, there was one patient who underwent laparoscopic retroperitoneal biopsy (not lymphadenectomy) for diagnosis of a lymph node metastasis (pN2) of contralateral upper tract TCC. The patient responded well on subsequent MVEC chemotherapy and open nephroureterectomy showed no evidence of residual tumor. This patient did not develop any port site metastasis. On the other hand, an inadequate preoperative diagnosis may represent a significant risk factor, because the operative technique might differ significantly.

Finally, it is important to mention that in all reported cases the retrieval of the specimen was carried out either without an organ bag ($n = 5$) or the bag was torn ($n = 1$). Therefore, retrieval of the specimen in an impermeable organ bag (i.e., LapSac) seems to be mandatory [81,82]. The fact that in all larger series except one [26] no port site metastases have been documented underlines the importance of surgical experience and technical expertise to minimize the risk of port site metastases.

Costs

To our knowledge, there are only a few studies concerning the comparison of costs of radical nephroureterectomy [83,84]. According to the model of cost analysis (Data 3.5 program, TreeAge software) proposed by Ogan et al. [85], the following factors have to be taken into account: equipment, personnel, operating time, medication, and hospital stay. In the study of the same group comparing laparoscopic versus open radical nephrectomy [84], the operating time did not differ dramatically, resulting in similar costs (US$2445 vs $2332); however, the equipment was more expensive for laparoscopy ($1122 vs $1809). On the other hand, laparoscopy required less cost for personnel ($1500 vs $1809), medication ($368 vs $739), and hospital stay ($1293 vs $2419). Particularly in Europe, these advantages (i.e., hospital stay) might be less dramatic; however, at our center at least, the equipment costs are considerably lower (i.e., mostly use of reusable instruments). The two-way analysis of Lotan and coworkers [83] revealed the operating time and hospital stay as the most important factors, mainly because they can still be reduced: for example, based on a hospital stay of 3 days, the operating time of laparoscopic radical prostatectomy has to be below 250 min to be more cost-effective than the open procedure. Meraney and Gill [84] were able to show that mainly by decreasing the operating time for radical nephroureterectomy, the laparoscopic approach became 12% more cost effective than open surgery. This may finally represent a significant breakthrough in favor of laparoscopic surgery, because economical reasons represent one of the major arguments against this technique.

Conclusion

There is no doubt that open radical nephroureterectomy still represents the gold standard for the management of upper tract transitional cell carcinoma. However, after more than 13 years, laparoscopic radical nephroureterectomy has withstood the test of time. Based on an evidence level of IIa (comparative studies, meta-analysis), the procedure offers all the advantages of minimally invasive surgery (less morbidity, earlier convalescence). At the centers of expertise worldwide, the learning curve has definitively plateaued and costs are at least similar to open surgery. The incidence of specific risks like port site metastases is low and can be further minimized by optimal preoperative diagnosis, careful intraoperative management (non-touch technique), and strict use of an organ bag for retrieval of the specimen. Based on this, the oncological outcome does not differ from the open technique. However, in cases of advanced tumors (pT3, N +) open surgery is still recommended.

References

1. Mazeman E (1976) Tumors of the upper urinary tract calyces, renal pelvis, and ureter. Eur Urol 2:120
2. Carr T, Powell PH, Ransden PE (1987) Nephroureterectomy. Br J Urol 59:99
3. Corrado F, Ferri C, Mannini D, Corrado G, Bertoni F, Bacchini P, Lelli G, Lieber MM, Song JM (1991) Transitional cell carcinoma of the upper urinary tract: evaluation of prognostic factors by histopathology and flow cytometric analysis. J Urol 145:1159–1163
4. Charbit L, Gendreau M-C, Mee S, Cukier J (1991) Tumors of the upper urinary tract: 10 years of experience. J Urol 146:1243–1246
5. Jurincic-Winkler C, Horlbeck R, Gasser A, Glenewinkel J, Klippel KF (1993) Urothelial cancer of the upper urinary tract. Urologe A 67:32
6. Tawfiek ER, Bagley DM (1997) Upper tract transitional cell carcinoma. Urology 50:321
7. Hall MC, Womack S, Sagalowsky AI, Carmody T, Erickstad MD, Roehrborn CG (1998) Prognostic factors, recurrence, and survival in transitional cell carcinoma of the upper urinary tract: a 30-year experience in 252 patients. Urology 52:594–601
8. Messing EM, Catalona W (1998) Urothelial tumors of the urinary tract. In: Walsh PC, Retik AB, Vaughan ED, Wein AJ (eds) Campbell's urology, 7th edn. Saunders, Philadelphia, pp 2327–2410
9. McDonald HP, Upchurch WE, Surdevant CE (1952) Nephroureterectomy—a new technique. J Urol 67:804
10. Clayman RV, Garske GL, Lange PH (1983) Total nephroureterectomy with ureteral intussusception and transureteral detachment and pull-through. Urology 21:482–486
11. Abercrombie GF, Eardley I, Payne SR, Walmsley BH, Vinnicombe J (1988) Modified nephroureterectomy. Long-term follow-up with particular reference to subsequent bladder tumors. Br J Urol 61:198–200
12. Bub P, Rassweiler J, Eisenberger F (1989) Ureteral stripping after transurethral circumscription of the orifice—an alternative of total surgical ureterectomy (English abstract). Akt Urol 20:67–69

13. Palou J, Caparros J, Orsola A, Xavier B, Vicente J (1995) Transurethral resection of the intramural ureter as the first step of nephroureterectomy. J Urol 154:43
14. Zubac DP, Kihl B (1997) One or two incisions for nephroureterectomy in transitional cell renal pelvis tumors. Scand J Urol 31:431–433
15. Angulo JC, Hontoria J, Sanchez-Chapado M (1998) One-incision nephroureterectomy endoscopically assisted transurethral stripping. Urology 52:203–207
16. Laguna MP, de la Rosette JJMCH (2001) The endoscopic approach to the distal ureter in nephroureterectomy for upper urinary tract tumor. J Urol 166:2017–2022
17. Salvador-Bayarri JS, Rodrigez-Villamil L, Imperatore V, Palou Redorta J, Villavicencio-Mavrich H, Vicente-Rodrigez J (2002) Bladder neoplasms after nephroureterectomy: does surgery of the lower ureter, transurethral resection or open surgery, influence the evolution? Eur Urol 41:30–33
18. Figenshau RS, Albala DM, Clayman RV, Kavoussi LR, Chandhoke P, Stone AM (1991) Laparoscopic nephrourectomy: initial laboratory experience. Min Invas Ther 1:93–97
19. Clayman RV, Kavoussi LR, Figenshau RS, Chandhoke P, Albala DM (1991) Laparoscopic nephroureterectomy: initial clinical case report. J Laparoendosc Surg 1:343–349
20. Chiu AW, Chen MT, Huang WJS, Juang GD, Lu SH, Chang LS (1992) Laparoscopic nephroureterectomy and endoscopic incision of bladder cuff. Min Invas Ther 1:299–303
21. Chirpaz A, Petibon E (1992) Nephro-ureterectomie gauche sous control coelioscopique. J Coelio-chir 2:32–34
22. Coptcoat MJ, Wickham JEA (1992) Laparoscopy in urology. Min Invas Ther 1:337
23. Rassweiler J, Henkel TO, Potempa DM, Coptcoat M, Alken P (1993) The technique of transperitoneal laparoscopic nephrectomy, adrenalectomy, and nephroureterectomy. Eur Urol 23:425
24. McDougall EM, Clayman RV, Elashry OM (1995) Laparoscopic nephroureterectomy for upper tract transitional cell cancer: Washington University experience. J Urol 154:975–980
25. Chung HJ, Chiu AW, Chen KK, Chang LS (1996) Retroperitoneoscopy-assisted nephroureterectomy for the management of upper tract urothelial cancer. Min Invas Ther 5:266
26. Barrett PH, Fentie DD, Taranger LA, Gonor SE, Weckworth PF, Visvanation K (1998) Laparoscopic assisted nephroureterectomy (TCC). J Endourol 12:S103
27. Keeley FX, Tolley DA (1998) Laparoscopic nephroureterectomy: making management of upper tract transitional-cell carcinoma entirely minimally invasive. J Endourol 12:139–141
28. Rassweiler J, Coptcoat M, Frede T (1999) Laparoscopic radical nephroureterectomy for treatment of renal cell and transitional cell carcinoma: Current status. Urol Integr Invest 4:225–237
29. Salomon L, Hoznek A, Cicco A, Gasman D, Chopin DK, Abbou CC (1999) Retroperitoneoscopic nephroureterectomy for renal pelvic tumors with a single iliac incision. J Urol 161:541–544
30. Shalhav AL, Dunn MD, Portis AJ, Elbahnashy AM, McDougall EM, Clayman RV (2000) Laparoscopic nephroureterectomy for upper tract transitional cell cancer: the Washington University experience. J Urol 163:1100–1104
31. McNeill SA, Chrisofos M, Tolley DA (2000) The long-term outcome after laparoscopic nephroureterectomy: a comparison with open nephroureterectomy. BJU Int 86:619–623

32. Gill IS, Sung GT, Hobart MG, Savage SJ, Meraney AM, Schweizer DK, Klein EA, Novick AC (2000) Laparoscopic radical nephroureterectomy for upper tract transitional cell carcinoma: the Cleveland Clinic experience. J Urol 164:1513–1522
33. Stifelman MD, Hyman MJ, Shichman S, Sosa RE (2001) Hand-assisted laparoscopic nephroureterectomy versus open nephroureterectomy for the treatment of transitional-cell carcinoma of the upper urinary tract. J Endourol 15:391–395
34. Seifman BD, Montie JE, Wolf JS Jr (2001) Prospective comparison between hand-assisted laparoscopic and open surgical nephroureterectomy for urothelial cell carcinoma. Urology 57:133
35. Jarrett TW, Chan DY, Cadeddu JA, Kavoussi LR (2001) Laparoscopic nephroureterectomy for the treatment of transitional cell carcinoma of the upper urinary tract. Urology 57:448–453
36. Chen J, Chueh SC, Hsu WT, Lai MK, Chen SC (2001) Modified approach of hand-assisted laparoscopic nephroureterectomy for transitional cell carcinoma of the upper urinary tract. Urology 58:930–934
37. Uozumi J, Fujiyama C, Meiri H, Tsukahara, T, Soejima C, Kanou T, Masaki Z (2002) Hand-assisted retroperitoneoscopic nephroureterectomy for upper urinary-tract urothelial tumors. J Endourol 16:743–747
38. Landman J, Lev RY, Bhayani S, Alberts G, Rehman J, Pattaras JG, Figenshau RS, Kibel AS, Clayman RV, McDougall EM (2002) Comparison of hand assisted and standard open nephroureterectomy for the management of localized transitional cell carcinoma. J Urol 167:2387–2391
39. Matsui Y, Ohara H, Icihoka K, Terada N, Yoshimura K, Terai A, Arai Y (2002) Retroperitoneoscopy-assisted total nephroureterectomy for upper urinary tract transitional cell carcinoma. Urology 60:1010–1015
40. Goel A, Hemal AK, Gupta NP (2002) Retroperitoneal laparoscopic radical nephrectomy and nephroureterectomy and comparison with open surgery. World J Urol 20:219–223
41. Wong C, Leveillee RJ (2002) Hand-assisted laparoscopic nephroureterectomy with cystoscopic en bloc excision of the distal ureter and bladder cuff. J Endourol 16:329–333
42. Kawauchi A, Fujiti A, Ukimura O, Yoneda K, Mizutani Y, Miki T (2003) Hand-assisted retroperitoneoscopic nephroureterectomy: comparison with the open procedure. J Urol 169:890–894
43. Schulze M, Seidensticker P, Frede T, Rassweiler J (2002) Laparoscopic radical nephroureterectomy for the treatment of transitional cell carcinoma of the kidney and ureter: an 8 year follow-up. Eur Urol 42 Suppl 1:139
44. Yoshino Y, Ono Y, Hattori R, Gotoh, M, Osamu K, Ohshima S (2003) Retroperitoneoscopic nephroureterectomy for transitional cell carcinoma of the renal pelvis and ureter: Nagoya experience. Urology 61:533–538
45. Klingler HC, Lodde M, Pycha A, Remzi M, Janetschek G, Marberger M (2003) Modified laparoscopic nephroureterectomy for treatment of upper urinary tract transitional cell cancer is not associated with increased risk of tumor recurrence. Eur Urol 44:442–447
46. Hattori R, Ono Y, Gotoh M, Yoshino Y, Ohshima S (2003) Retroperitoneoscopic nephroureterectomy for transitional cell carcinoma of the renal pelvis and ureter: Nagoya experience. J Urol 169:77 (Suppl, abstract No. 299)
47. Bariol SV, Stewart GD, McNeill SA, Tolley DA (2004) Oncological control following laparoscopic nephroureterectomy: 7-year outcome. J Urol 172:1805–1808

48. El Fettouh HA, Rassweiler JJ, Schulze M, Salomon L, Allan J, Ramakumar S, Jarrett T, Abbou CC, Tolley DA, Kavoussi LR, Gill IS (2002) Laparoscopic radical nephroureterectomy: results of an international multicenter study. Eur Urol 42:447–452
49. Doublet JD, Janetschek G, Joyce A, Mandressi A, Rassweiler J, Tolley D (2002) Nephroureterectomy: guideline recommendations. Guidelines Laparoscopy, EAU-Guidelines, p. 21
50. Rassweiler J, Henkel TO, Stock C, Greschner M, Becker P, Preminger GM, Schulman CC, Frede T, Alken P (1994) Retroperitoneal laparoscopic nephrectomy and other procedures in the upper retroperitoneum using a balloon dissection technique. Eur Urol 25:229
51. Rassweiler JJ, Seemann O, Frede T, Henkel TO, Alken P (1998) Retroperitoneoscopy: Experience with 200 cases. J Urol 160:1265–1269
52. Gill IS, Rassweiler JJ (1999) Retroperitoneal renal surgery: our approach. Urology 54:734–738
53. Rassweiler J, Frede T, Henkel TO, Stock C, Alken P (1998) Nephrectomy: a comparative study between the transperitoneal and retroperitoneal laparoscopic versus the open approach. Eur Urol 13:489–496
54. Rassweiler J, Fornara P, Weber M, Janetschek G, Fahlenkamp D, Henkel T, Beer M, Stackl W, Boeckmann W, Recker F, Lampel A, Fischer C, Humke U, Miller K (1998) Laparoscopic nephrectomy: the experience of the laparoscopic working group of the German Urological Association. J Urol 160:18–21
55. Elbahnasy AM, Hoenig DM, Shalav A, McDougall EM, Clayman RV (1998) Laparoscopic staging of bladder tumor: concerns about port site metastases. J Endourol 12:55–59
56. Rassweiler J, Tsivian A, Ravi Kumar AV, Lymberakis C, Schulze M, Seemann O, Frede T (2003) Oncological safety of laparoscopic surgery for urological malignancies: experience with more than 1,000 operations. J Urol 169:2072–2075
57. Lee BR, Jabbour ME, Marshall FF, Smith AD, Jarrett TW (1999) 13-year survival comparison of percutaneous and open nephroureterectomy approaches for management of transitional cell carcinoma of renal collecting system: equivalent outcomes. J Endourol 13:289
58. Wolf S, Moon TD, Madisom WI, Nakada SY (1998) Hand-assisted laparoscopic nephrectomy: comparison to standard laparoscopic nephrectomy. J Urol 160:22–27
59. Steinberg JR, Matin SF (2004) Laparoscopic radical nephroureterectomy: dilemma of the distal ureter. Curr Opin Urol 14:61–65
60. Hetherington JW, Ewing R, Philip NH (1986) Modified nephroureterectomy: a risk of tumor implantation. Br J Urol 58:368–370
61. Jones DR, Moisey CU (1993) A cautionary tale of the modified "pluck" nephroureterectomy. Br J Urol 71:486
62. Arango O, Bielsa O, Carles J, Gelabert-Mas A (1997) Massive tumor implantation in the endoscopic resected area in modified nephroureterectomy, J Urol 157:1839
63. Pascual Regueiro D, Garcia de Jalon Martinez A, Sanch Serrano C, Mallen Mateo E, Blas Marin M, Rioja Sanz LA (2003) Tumor recurrence in the resected area of the ureteral meatus after endoscopic disinsertion during radical nephroureterectomy (English abstract). Actas Urol Esp 27:308–311
64. Baughman SM, Sexton W, Bishoff JT (2003) Multiple intravesical linear staples identified during surveillance cystoscopy after laparoscopic nephroureterectomy. Urology 62:351

65. Komatsu H, Tanabe N, Kubodera S, Maezawa H, Ueno A (1997) The role of lymphadenectomy in the treatment of transitional cell carcinoma of the upper urinary tract. J Urol 157:1622
66. Miyake H, Hara I, Gohji K, Arakawa S, Kamidono S (1998) The significance of lymphadenectomy in transitional cell carcinoma of the upper urinary tract. Br J Urol 82:494
67. Portis AJ, Yan Y, Landman J, Chen C, Barrett PH, Fentie DD, Ono Y, McDougall EM, Clayman RV (2002) Long-term follow-up after laparoscopic radical nephrectomy. J Urol 167:1257–1262
68. Cicco A, Salomon L, Hoznek H, Alame W, Saint F, Bralet MB, Antiphon P, Chopin DK, Abbou CC (2000) Carcinological risks and retroperitoneal laparoscopy. Eur Urol 38:606–612
69. Ahmed, I, Shaikh, NA, Kapadia, CR (1998) Track recurrence of renal pelvic transitional cell carcinoma after laparoscopic nephrectomy. Br J Urol 81:319
70. Otani M, Irie S, Tsuji Y (1999) Port site metastasis after laparoscopic nephrectomy: unsuspected transitional cell carcinoma within a tuberculous atrophic kidney. J Urol 162:486
71. Ong AM, Bhayani SB, Pavlovich CP (2003) Trocar site recurrence after laparoscopic nephroureterectomy. J Urol 170:1301
72. Matsui Y, Ohara H, Ichioka K, Terada N, Yoshimura K, Terai A (2004) Abdominal wall metastasis after retroperitoneoscopic assisted total nephroureterectomy for renal pelvic cancer. J Urol 171:793
73. Naderi N, Nieuwenhuijzen JA, Bex A, Kooistra A, Horenblas S (2004) Port site metastasis after laparoscopic nephro-ureterectomy for transitional cell carcinoma. Eur Urol 46:440–441
74. Bangma CH, Kirkels WJ, Chada S, Schröder FH (1995) Cutaneous metastasis following laparoscopic lymphadenectomy for prostatic carcinoma. J Urol 153:1635–1636
75. Andersen JR, Steven K (1995) Implantation metastasis after laparoscopic biopsy of bladder cancer. J Urol 153:1047–1048
76. Doret M, Mege JL, Fendler JP, Kepenekian G (2001) Parietal metastasis in nephrectomy track reveals pyelic transitional cell carcinoma. J Urol 165:520
77. Sharma NK, Nicol A, Powell CS (1994) Track infiltration following percutaneous resection of renal pelvic transitional cell carcinoma. Br J Urol 73:597–598
78. Yamada Y, Kobayashi Y, Yao A, Amamaka K, Takechi Y, Umezu K (2002) Nephrostomy tract tumor seeding following percutaneous manipulation of a renal pelvic carcinoma (English abstract). Hinyoikika Kiyo 48:415–418
79. Treuthardt C, Dannuser H, Studer UE (2004) Tumor seeding following percutaneous antegrade management of transitional cell carcinoma in the renal pelvis. Eur Urol 46:442–443
80. Slywotzky C, Maya M (1994) Needle tract seeding of transitional cell carcinoma following fine-needle aspiration of renal mass. Abdom Imaging 19:174–176
81. Urban DA, Kerbl K, McDougall EM, Stone AM, Fadden PT, Clayman RV (1993) Organ entrapment and renal morcellation: permeability studies. J Urol 150:1792
82. Rassweiler J, Stock C, Frede T, Seemann O, Alken P (1998) Organ retrieval systems for endoscopic nephrectomy: a comparative study. J Endourol 12:325–333
83. Lotan Y, Gettman MT, Roehrborn CG, Pearle MS, Cadeddu J (2002) Cost comparison for laparoscopic and open nephrectomy: analysis of individual parameters. Urology 59:821

84. Meraney AM, Gill IS (2002) Financial analysis of open versus laparoscopic radical nephrectomy and nephroureterectomy. J Urol 167:1757–1762
85. Ogan K, Lotan Y, Koeneman K, Perale MS, Caddedu JA, Rassweiler J (2002) Laparoscopic versus open retroperitoneal lymph node dissection: a cost analysis. J Urol 168:1945; discussion 1949

Hand-Assisted Retroperitoneoscopic Nephroureterectomy

Akihiro Kawauchi, Akira Fujito, Kimihiko Yoneda, Jintetsu Soh, Yasuyuki Naitoh, Osamu Ukimura, Yoichi Mizutani, and Tsuneharu Miki

Summary. In laparoscopic operations for upper urinary tract transitional cell carcinoma (TCC), three kinds of approach, the transperitoneal, retroperitoneal, and hand-assisted transperitoneal, have been reported. We have performed hand-assisted retroperitoneoscopic nephroureterectomy (HALS) since 2000. The surgical techniques and the operative results of 61 cases of HALS are described and analyzed. These procedures were effective and safe for upper urinary tract TCC.

Keywords. Laparoscopy, Hand-assisted retroperitoneoscopic nephroureterectomy, Upper urinary tract, Transitional cell carcinoma

Introduction

Hand-assisted techniques for renal surgery have been reported using the transperitoneal approach since 1994 [1,2]. Although the advantages and disadvantages of hand assistance have been much discussed, this technique has already been established for the surgeon as an alternative choice [3–6]. It is especially useful when the large parenchymatous organs such as the kidney are removed intact or when surgeons feel difficulty using standard laparoscopic procedures. On the other hand, the retroperitoneal approach for renal surgery has been used mainly for benign lesions and as the surgeon's choice for malignant lesions [7,8]. Generally it is recognized as the approach in which complications of intra-abdominal organs are rare and difficulties due to previous intra-abdominal operations are few, although the operating space is restricted.

We have been developing hand-assisted retroperitoneoscopic radical nephrectomy since 1999 and have performed hand-assisted retroperitoneoscopic nephroureterectomy (HALS) since 2000 [9,10]. In reports comparing these with

Department of Urology, Kyoto Prefectural University of Medicine, Kawaramachi-Hirokoji, Kyoto 602-8566, Japan open procedures, not only were wounds smaller but there were also many other advantages such as reduction of blood loss, less pain, and fewer days to full recovery. Here we present our recent techniques and the operative results of HALS.

Technique

Preoperatively, the number and anatomical position of the renal vessels were assessed by magnetic resonance imaging angiography or three-dimensional computed tomography. A laxative was prescribed the evening before surgery and a glycerin enema was performed on the morning of the operation day.

The patients were placed in the lateral position with a compression stocking and an antithrombus instrument on the legs. The operating table was flexed to maximize the space between the 12th rib and the iliac crest, and was rotated if necessary. A 7.0–7.5-cm incision was made on the lower abdomen as described in Fig. 1 beneath the lower limit of the umbilicus. The anterior and posterior fascias of the rectus muscle were incised and the retroperitoneal space was dissected bluntly with fingers, forceps, and retractors. After the Gerota's fascia and the psoas muscle were exposed under direct vision, the ureter was identified and ligated to avoid distal migration of tumor cells via the urine. The LAP DISC (Hakko Shoji, Tokyo, Japan) was placed at the incision. A 12-mm port was inserted through the LAP DISC and a pneumoretroperitoneum was created at 12 mmHg with carbon dioxide. Two 12-mm trocars were inserted, one dorsally and the other centrally, under direct vision from the port introduced through the LAP DISC. The 12-mm port that had been placed through the LAP DISC was removed and used as a third trocar. The occluding ring of the LAP DISC was tightened and the 12 mmHg pneumoretroperitoneum was re-established. The third trocar was placed under vision from the first port. Port placement is shown in Fig. 1.

The assistant's hand, the left for the right kidney and the right for the left kidney, was inserted through the LAP DISC (Fig. 2), and intraretroperitoneal pressure was changed to 8–10 mmHg. The hand is mainly used for palpation of the renal artery in order to identify it quickly, for retraction of the kidney, and

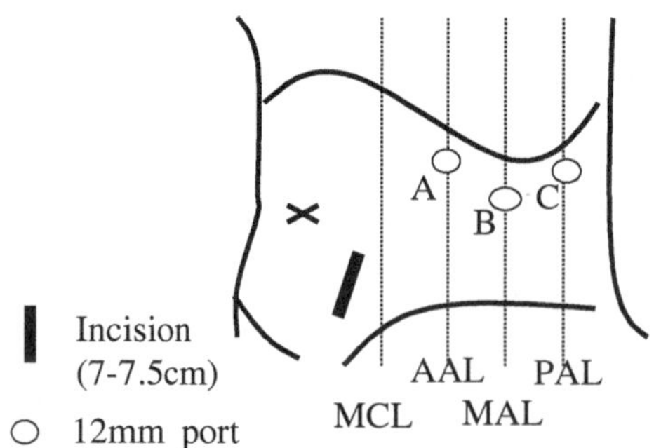

Fig. 1. Port placement. *A*, 12 mm trocar; *B*, 12 mm trocar (laparoscope); *C*, 12 mm trocar. *PAL*, posterior axillary line; *MAL*, mid-axillary line; *AAL*, anterior axillary line; *MCL*, mid-clavicular line. *Bold line*, 7.0–7.5 cm incision for hand insertion

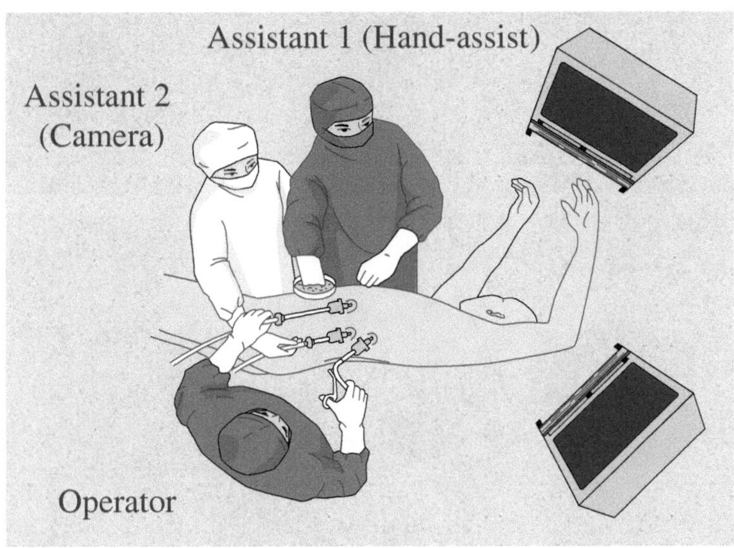

FIG. 2. The positions of operator and assistants for nephrectomy. The operator stands behind the patient's back, while the two assistants stand on the other side. One assistant inserts his hand through the LAP DISC

for blunt dissection around the kidney. A 10-mm 0-degree laparoscope was inserted through the central trocar.

Generally a space between the ureter and the aorta or the vena cava was easily created by a finger. The laterocornal fascia, which covers the lateral side of the ureter, was nipped by the fingers and cut by ultrasonic scissors with finger assistance to the diaphragm. The posterior part of the Gerota's fascia was easily dissected using the hand. The ureter was identified near the lower pole and the assistant was able to palpate the aorta on the left or the vena cava on the right at the lateral side of the ureter. Usually the renal artery was immediately identified by palpation. The renal artery was dissected, secured by ligature clips, and transected with scissors. Located anteriorly, the renal vein was identified and dissected. On the left side the gonadal vein and the lumbar vein were transected. The renal pedicle was held and retracted easily and quickly by two fingers. This retraction made it easy to handle an endoscopic gastrointestinal anastomosis vascular stapler. The renal vein was secured and transected with this instrument. The adrenal gland was usually preserved. The posterior and anterior aspects of the kidney were dissected with the fingers and/or ultrasonic scissors. Blunt dissection around the kidney was quick and easy in all cases. After dissecting the upper pole of the kidney without the adrenal gland, circumferential mobilization of the kidney was completed.

The patient was changed to the lithotomy position. If there was no tumor in the intramural ureter or if the tumor did not extend into the bladder, ureterec-

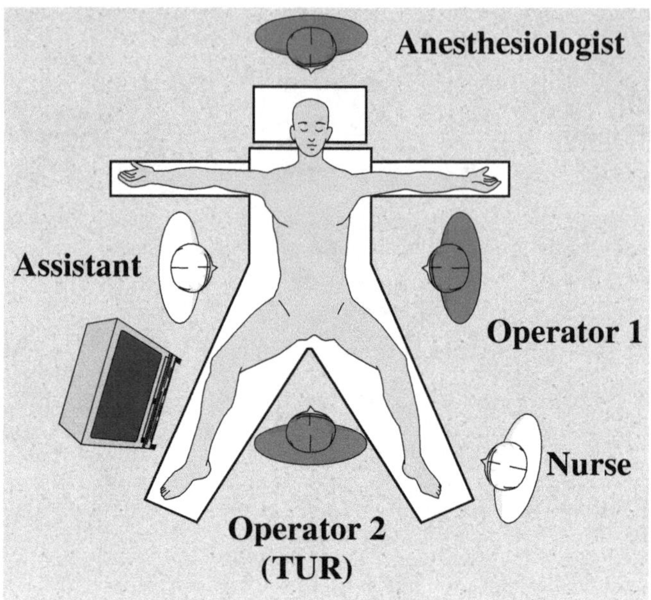

Fig. 3. The positions of operator and assistants for lower ureterectomy. Ureterectomy and transurethral excision of the bladder cuff and the intramural ureter were performed at the same time by two operators. *TUR*, transurethral resection

tomy and transurethral excision of the bladder cuff and the intramural ureter were performed at the same time by two separate operators (Fig. 3). Generally ureterectomy was performed through the 7–7.5-cm pararectal incision in which the hand had been inserted. When dissection of the lower ureter was difficult, the incision was extended 2–5 cm.

In this procedure the kidney was pulled out from the incision, and the connected ureter was retracted and dissected toward the bladder. At the same time, the other operator performed transurethral excision of the bladder cuff and the intramural ureter. The excision was completed until just before extravesical fat tissue was confirmed circumferentially, then the irrigation fluid was replaced by CO_2 gas in order to prevent dissemination of tumor cells in the extravesical region by the irrigation fluid itself. After ureterectomy with the bladder cuff was completed by dissection from the incision, the specimen was extracted intact through the LAP DISC. The bladder defect was repaired by two or three sutures using absorbable suture. A Foley indwelling catheter was inserted for 3–7 days and removed after a cystogram confirmed there was no leakage.

In cases in which there was a tumor in the intramural ureter or the tumor extended into the bladder, ureterectomy and partial cystectomy were performed by conventional open method after a 2–5 cm elongation of the incision.

Results

The indications were renal pelvic tumors with a lower stage than T3 N0 M0 and ureteral tumors with a lower stage than T2N0M0. Since 2000, HALS has been performed in 61 patients. The operating time was defined as the elapsed time from first incision to final closure minus the time for the change from the lateral to the lithotomy position, which was 30min on average. Mean operating time and insufflation time were 236 and 128min, respectively. The mean time between starting the ureterectomy and the end of wound closure was 78min. The mean estimated blood loss was 250ml.

The complication and open conversion rates were 8% (5/61) and 2% (1/61), respectively. In one patient, bleeding from surrounding fatty tissue and the left adrenal gland was found after completion of nephrectomy. When we tried to stop the bleeding laparoscopically, the bleeding point could not be located. Consequently the bleeding was stopped by open conversion with a 10-cm elongation of the wound. Total blood loss was 1500ml. Other postoperative complications were pneumothorax in one case and wound infection in three cases. The pneumothorax was diagnosed as spontaneous because it was observed on the side opposite to the operation.

Histological examination revealed transitional cell carcinoma (TCC) in 61 cases. The mean follow-up period was 22 months and the recurrence rate was 36% (22/61). Bladder recurrence without metastasis was found in 17 patients, while metastases were found in five patients including lung, liver, and lymph node with or without bladder recurrence. No port site or incisional site recurrences were found. The disease-free survival rate in 49 cases that were followed up for at least for 6 months was compared with that in 47 open surgery cases. There were no significant differences between the two groups (Fig. 4).

Discussion

This procedure has the characteristics of both hand-assisted surgery and the retroperitoneal approach for the kidney. The standard transperitoneal hand-assisted procedure has been reported frequently. In retroperitoneal hand assistance the working space opened by the hand was more than we expected, although the retroperitoneal space is still small compared to the peritoneal cavity. On the other hand, it is possible but difficult for the operator to use his own hand, since the space is barely sufficient for flexible movements. Accordingly an assistant's hand is used in this procedure. The disadvantage of this kind of hand assistance was thought to be that the coordination between the assistant's hand and the operator's forceps was inferior to that in the reported hand-assisted laparoscopic procedure in which the operator inserted his own hand. Also, the operator has to be careful of causing burn injury to the assistant's hand by electrocautery or from the ultrasonic scissors. The advantage was thought to be that the dissection was finer than in the hand-assisted laparoscopic procedure,

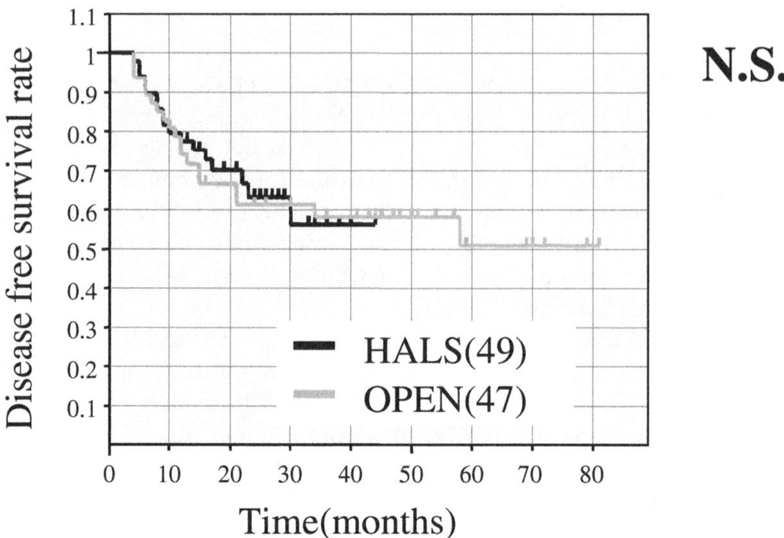

Fig. 4. Disease-free survival rates in hand-assisted retroperitoneoscopic and open nephroureterectomy. *N.S.*, not significant; *HALS*, hand-assisted retroperitoneoscopic nephroureterectomy

since the operator was able to use both hands for forceps or scissors as in standard laparoscopic surgery. The retroperitoneal hand-assisted approach for nephrectomy is also useful as an educational procedure. In an analysis of the learning curve of the approach for nephrectomy performed by 18 less experienced urologists [11], the insufflation time in the fourth or previous cases was significantly longer than that in cases 16 and later. In case numbers 5–10 the insufflation time was 14–24 min longer than that in case number 16 and later. In this approach for nephrectomy, 5–10 cases were necessary for less-experienced urologists to gain average operating skills. Accordingly, it may be reasonable for less-experienced surgeons to begin standard laparoscopic procedures after experiencing 10 cases using this approach. Thus, this approach is useful as a first step in laparoscopic nephrectomy.

The advantages of the retroperitoneal approach for retroperitoneal organs have been mentioned in many papers [12]. The potential for intraperitoneal contamination with cancer cells is eliminated. Urinoma or seroma collections remain restricted to the retroperitoneal space. The nonmanipulation of the bowel leads to minimal paralytic ileus. Furthermore, previous intra-abdominal operations might not negatively influence the retroperitoneal procedure [9]. Of course, for cases with a history of previous retroperitoneal operation, such as surgery for urinary stone, the transabdominal approach may be easier.

The approach to the distal ureter and the bladder cuff is one of the most important points of laparoscopic nephroureterectomy. The distal ureter and the bladder cuff must be removed completely without tumor seeding. Moreover, minimally invasive aspects such as the smaller wound and the shorter operating time are characteristic of the laparoscopic procedure. Several approaches have been reported in this regard [12–15]. The advantages of our procedure are that removal of the bladder cuff and suturing of the bladder rent are secure through the 7.0-cm incision without the necessity of any additional ports [10]. The operating time is reduced by the method of performing the ureterectomy and transurethral excision simultaneously. We also take precautions against tumor spillage by ligation of the ureter as early as possible, bladder lavage before the transurethral procedure, and replacement of irrigated fluid with CO_2 gas just before perforation of the bladder wall.

In our previous study, the operative results were superior to those in the open procedure [10]. On the other hand, the results also compare favorably to those of other series [12–22]. The published data on laparoscopic or retroperitoneoscopic nephroureterectomy with or without hand-assistance were reviewed and compared with the present series (Table 1). Regarding complications, the rate of 8% in the present series was lower than the rates in other standard laparoscopic series, while those in other hand-assisted series were similar. Seifman et al. commented that hand assistance maintains the benefits of laparoscopy in terms of

Table 1. Comparison of laparoscopic nephroureterectomy reports

First author	Keeley	Shalhav	Jarrett	Gill	Stifelman	Hsueh	Present study
Reference	[18]	[19]	[20]	[12]	[16]	[22]	
No. of patients	22	25	25	42	22	58	61
Technique	TP	TP	TP	RP	TP-HALS	RP-HALS	RP-HALS
Distal ureter	TUR	Stapled	Stapled	Transvesical technique	Transvesical technique	Open	Transurethral excision + open at the same time
Mean operating time (min)	2.6	7.7	5.5	3.9	4.5	4.3	3.9
Mean blood loss (ml)	—	199	440	242	180	409	250
% Complications	—	48	36	12	5	3	8
% Open conversion	18	0	4	5	0	0	2
% Recurrence	9	52	68[a]	26	27	19	36
Mean follow-up (months)	—	39	—	11.1	13	16.1	22

TP, transperitoneal; RP, retroperitoneal; HALS, hand-assisted retroperitoneoscopic nephroureterectomy; TUR, transurethral resection.

[a] Concurrent bladder tumors are included.

patient convalescence while technically simplifying the procedure for the surgeon [17]. Our data support their impression.

With regard to cancer control, the recurrence rates of 36% in our series are comparable to those in previous reports of laparoscopic operations [12,16,19,20]. In long-term cancer control, there were no significant differences in 5-year metastasis-free survival rates between the transperitoneal standard laparoscopic and the open approach [21]. However, an extended follow-up including morbidity will be necessary to assess the true efficacy of this procedure.

In conclusion, hand-assisted retroperitoneoscopic nephroureterectomy is an effective and safe procedure for upper urinary tract transitional cell carcinoma. However, the influence of hand assistance on tumor spillage or distant dissemination is unclear. Longer follow-up will be necessary to assess the efficacy of this procedure.

References

1. Tierney JP, Oliver SR, Kusminsky RE, Tiley EH, Boland JP (1994) Laparoscopic radical nephrectomy with intra-abdominal manipulation. Min Invas Ther 3:303–305
2. Nakada SY, Moon TD, Gist M, Mahvi D (1997) Use of the Pneumo Sleeve as an adjunct in laparoscopic nephrectomy. Urology 49:612–623
3. Wolf JS Jr, Moon TD, Nakada SY (1998) Hand-assisted laparoscopic nephrectomy: comparison to standard laparoscopic nephrectomy. J Urol 160:22
4. Batler RA, Campbell SC, Funk JT, Gonzalez CM, Nadler RB (2001) Hand-assisted vs. retroperitoneal laparoscopic nephrectomy. J Endourol 15:899–902
5. Wolf JS Jr (2001) Hand-assisted laparoscopy: pro. Urology 58:310
6. Gill IS (2001) Hand-assisted laparoscopy: con. Urology 58:313
7. Gaur DD, Agarwal DK, Purohit KC (1993) Retroperitoneal laparoscopic nephrectomy. Initial case report. J Urol 149:103–105
8. Gill IS, Meraney AM, Schweizer DK, Savage SS, Hobart MG, Sung GT, Nelson D, Novick AC (2001) Laparoscopic radical nephrectomy in 100 patients. Cancer 92:1843–1855
9. Kawauchi A, Fujito A, Ukimura O, Soh J, Mizutani Y, Imaide Y, Miki T (2002) Hand assisted retroperitoneoscopic radical nephrectomy: initial experience. Int J Urol 9: 480–484
10. Kawauchi A, Fujito A, Ukimura O, Yoneda K, Mizutani Y, Miki T (2003) Hand-assisted retroperitoneoscopic nephroureterectomy: comparison to open procedure. J Urol 169:890–894
11. Kawauchi A, Fujito A, Soh J, Yoneda K, Ukimura O, Mizutani Y, Miki T (2005) Learning curve of hand-assisted retroperitoneoscopic nephrectomy in less-experienced laparoscopic surgeons. Int J Urol, 12, 1–6
12. Gill IS, Sung GT, Hobart MG, Savage SJ, Meraney AM, Schweizer DK, Klein EA, Novick AC (2000) Laparoscopic radical nephroureterectomy for upper tract transitional cell carcinoma: the Cleveland Clinic experience. J Urol 164:1513–1522
13. Salomon L, Hoznek A, Cicco A, Gasman D, Chopin DK, Abbou CC (1999) Retroperitoneoscopic nephroureterectomy for renal pelvic tumors with a single iliac incision. J Urol 161:541–549
14. Landman J, Lev RY, Bhayani S, Alerts G, Rehman J, Pattaras JG, Figenshau RS, Kibel AS, Clayman RJ, McDougall E (2002) Comparison of hand assisted and standard

laparoscopic radical nephroureterectomy for the management of localized transitional cell carcinoma. J Urol 167:2387–2391
15. Gonzalez CM, Batler RA, Schoor RA, Hairston JC, Nadler RB (2001) A novel endoscopic approach towards resection of the distal ureter with surrounding bladder cuff during hand assisted laparoscopic nephroureterectomy. J Urol 165:483–485
16. Stifelman MD, Sosa RE, Andrade A, Tarantino A, Shichman SJ (2000) Hand-assisted laparoscopic nephroureterectomy for the treatment of transitional cell carcinoma of the upper urinary tract. Urology 56:741–747
17. Seifman BD, Montie JE, Wolf JS Jr (2001) Prospective comparison between hand-assisted laparoscopic and open surgical nephroureterectomy for urothelial cell carcinoma. Urology 57:133
18. Keeley FX, Tolley DA (1998) Laparoscopic nephroureterectomy: making management of upper-tract transitional cell carcinoma entirely minimally invasive. J Endourol 12:139
19. Shalhav AL, Dunn MD, Portis AJ, Elbahnasy AM, McDougall EM, Clayman RT (2000) Laparoscopic nephroureterectomy for upper tract transitional cell cancer: the Washington University experience. J Urol 163:1100–1104
20. Jarrett TW, Chan DY, Cadeddu JA, Kavoussi LR (2001) Laparoscopic nephroureterectomy for the treatment of transitional cell carcinoma of the upper urinary tract. Urology 57:448–453
21. Bariol SV, Stewart GD, McNeill SA, Tolley DA (2004) Oncological control following laparoscopic nephroureterectomy: 7-year outcome. J Urol 172:1805–1808
22. Hsueh TY, Huang YH, Chiu AW, Shen KH, Lee YH (2004) A comparison of the clinical outcome between open and hand-assisted laparoscopic nephroureterectomy for upper urinary tract transitional cell carcinoma. BJU Int 94:798–201

Part 3
Urinary Bladder

Laparoscopic Radical Cystectomy and Urinary Diversion

Osamu Ukimura and Inderbir S. Gill

Summary. Most reported publications regarding laparoscopic radical cystectomy (LRC) have focused on technical feasibility and perioperative outcomes of the institutions' initial experiences. Subsequent construction of urinary diversion remains a challenging procedure. Recent increasing experience from major medical centers worldwide indicates rising interest and expertise in LRC. We describe the histological and experimental background, surgical technique, surgical outcomes, and future directions of LRC and urinary diversion.

Keywords. Laparoscopy, Radical cystectomy, Bladder cancer, Urinary diversion

Introduction

With worldwide acceptance of laparoscopic surgery, minimally invasive surgery has moved into the mainstream of urology surgery. Laparoscopic procedures have currently expanded for treatment of cancer in the pelvic organs. Although radical cystectomy is the accepted standard for treatment of patients with localized muscle invasive bladder cancer, open radical cystectomy with orthotopic urinary diversion is a major demanding surgery for patients, involving long postoperative recovery. A natural progression has been made to applying the laparoscopic technique to bladder surgery, because of its potential advantages in decreased blood loss, less postoperative pain, early return to full activity, and better cosmesis. Although the most challenging aspect of laparoscopic surgery is reconstructive procedures, Gill and colleagues recently reported initial laparoscopic radical cystectomy (LRC) with either ileal conduit or orthotopic urinary diversion in patients with muscle invasive bladder cancer, with entire procedure being performed purely intracorporeally [1,2]. In this chapter, we review the current experience with LRC and urinary diversion, focusing on histological and

Section of Laparoscopic and Robotic Surgery, Glickman Urological Institute, A100, The Cleveland Clinic Foundation, 9500 Euclid Avenue, Cleveland, OH 44195, USA

experimental background, controversies, surgical technique, surgical outcomes, and future directions.

Historical and Experimental Background

In early 1992, Parra et al. described the initial report of laparoscopic simple cystectomy, in a paraplegic woman suffering from recurrent pyocystis of retained bladder who had already undergone open surgical urinary diversion a few months earlier [3]. In 1995, Sanchez et al. reported the first case of laparoscopic assisted radical cystectomy with an ileal conduit performed extracorporeally in a woman with invasive bladder cancer [4].

Feasible laparoscopic options of the common urinary diversions have been demonstrated by early clinical experience or well-designed studies of experimental animal models. Kozminski and Partamian performed the first laparoscopically assisted ileal conduit construction, with the bowel anastomosis and both Bricker ureteroileal anastomoses performed extracorporeally through extended port sites [5]. Anderson et al. evaluated the feasibility of laparoscopic-assisted Mainz II (sigmoid-rectum) pouch in nine pigs; the cystectomy and dissection of ureter and large bowel were performed laparoscopically, and the Mainz II pouch was created extracorporeally [6].

Although the authors cited above established laparoscopic feasibility of certain portions of laparoscopic cystectomy or urinary diversion, it was not until 2000 that entire LRC and completely intracorporeal ileal conduit urinary diversion was employed clinically in two patients with bladder cancer, following a successful pilot experimental study in an animal model (10 pigs) by the author's institution [1,7]. Similarly, in the Cleveland Clinic the completely intracorporeal construction of orthotopic ileal neobladder (Studer) was initially developed successfully in an animal model (12 pigs), followed by clinical application of orthotopic urinary diversion in two patients and an Indiana pouch in one [2,8]. In 2000, Turk et al. reported LRC with a Mainz II pouch entirely intracorporeally in five patients [9]. These purely intracorporeal laparoscopic procedures duplicated principles of open surgery, and demonstrated that reconstruction of the bowel could be performed with purely intracorporeal freehand suturing techniques without anastomosis strictures or leak on follow-up [1,2,9]. Indications for choosing the type of laparoscopic urinary diversion that is best suited to a patient are not different from those of open surgery.

There is considerable validity to the advantages of purely laparoscopic techniques offered by the major academic centers, although creation of urinary diversion using purely intracorporeal suturing techniques is likely considered as technically challenging during the early learning experience, resulting in the requirement of longer operative times. Recent increasing interest in open-assisted creation of urinary diversion following LRC may indicate a trend to facilitate the broader expansion of LRC into the urology community worldwide, in a transition toward being given the full benefits through minimally invasive purely intracorporeal procedures.

Surgical Technique

Patient selection for LRC involves those with organ-confined, muscle-invasive, non-bulky bladder cancer as determined by preoperative radiological and clinical evaluations. Current exclusion criteria consist of histories of prior radiotherapy and neoadjuvant chemotherapy, or morbidly obese patients, because of the potential increase of technical challenge. In relatively obese patients, difficulty may be anticipated in pulling a loop of bowel through an obese abdominal wall to the skin level. Prior abdominal surgery is only a relative contraindication, although attention must be paid to avoid injury upon insertion of the initial laparoscopic access.

Surgical techniques of LRC aim to mirror established open radical cystectomy. Laparoscopic radical cystectomy typically requires a transperitoneal 5- or 6-port technique [1,2]. Briefly: (1) Peritoneal incision starts in the midline in the rectovesical pouch (with division of vasa deferentia, followed by incision of Denonvilliers fascia), and extending up to the common iliac artery in either side at the point of identifying crossing of the ureter; then, carried distally along the external iliac vessels up to the pubic bone, followed by its extension anteriorly with inverted V-shaped peritoneotomy. (2) Control of the lateral and posterior vascular pedicles of the bladder and prostate is achieved using the Endo-GIA stapler (U. S. Surgical, Norwalk, CT, USA). (3) Both ureters are mobilized, clipped (facilitating its hydrostatic distension), and divided close to the bladder (evaluating the distal ureteral margin for frozen section). (4) After developing the retropubic space, in similar fashion to laparoscopic radical prostatectomy, attachments of the prostate are released, and the radical cystoprostatectomy specimen is entrapped in an Endocatch-II bag (US Surgical, Norwalk, CT, USA), with the entire perivesical fat being maintained. In the female, a sponge stick in the vagina or Koh colpotomizer system (Cooper Surgical, Trumbull, CT, USA) facilitates the vaginal apex to be identified. The specimens (including prostate in men; uterus/fallopian tube/ovary in women) can be retrieved either through the vagina, a midline 5-cm incision, or rectum (in considering Mainz II in the next step).

Following LRC, extended lymphadenectomy is performed to achieve clearance of lymphatic tissues by skeletonizing following anatomy bilaterally, genitofemoral nerve, external iliac artery, external iliac vein, obturator nerve, hypogastric artery, common iliac artery, and pubic bone [10].

Currently, no universal approach is established for the reconstructive urinary diversion. The urinary diversions can be performed purely intracorporeally (as described below), or in open-assisted fashion. Urinary diversions consist of either noncontinent urinary diversion (ileal conduit, cutaneous ureterostomy, or incontinent ileovesicostomy,) or continent urinary diversion (orthotopic ileal neobladder, Mainz II pouch, or catheterizable reservoir). An ileal loop or orthotopic ileal neobladder seem preferable options.

Purely Laparoscopic Ileal Conduit [1]

Isolation of the ileal loop (15 cm segment with 15 cm proximal to the ileocecal junction), division of mesentery, and restoring bowel continuity are performed with an Endo-GIA stapler (using 3.5-mm blue cartridge for ileum and 2.5-mm gray vascular cartridge for mesentery; additionally the transected ends of the ileum oversewn with running 2-0 Vicryl for added security). The left ureter is delivered retroperitoneally to the right under the sigmoid mesocolon. Creation of the ileal stoma at a preoperatively marked site facilitates intracorporeal suturing of the ureteroileal anastomosis by providing a fixation for the ileal segment. After spatulating the ureteral cut edge, a continuous suture (4-0 Vicryl, RB-1 needle) is performed in 80% of the posterior (far) wall, followed by passing the 6-F J-stent (that was already inserted into the conduit lumen) into the ureter up to the renal pelvis. After completion of anastomosis for remainder of the posterior wall, the anterior (near) wall of anastomosis is completed with a separate running suture.

Purely Laparoscopic Orthotopic Ileal Neobladder [2]

Isolation of the ileal loop (55–65 cm segment with 15 cm proximal to the ileocecal junction), division of the mesentery, and restoration of bowel continuity are performed with an Endo-GIA stapler as described above. With the proximal 10-cm length ileum maintained intact (unopened) for the Studer limb, the remaining distal segment 45–55 cm long is opened along its antimesenteric border, following the gentle irrigation of bowel lumen by a laparoscopic suction irrigator.

The posterior plate of the pouch is created by a continuous intracorporeal suture (2-0 Vicryl, CT-1 needle). In closing the anterior plate partially, the most caudal part of the anterior plate is selected for a hole 8 mm in diameter for urethra-neovesical anastomosis, where running 2-0 Vicryl sutures on a UR-6 needle are placed. Before the completion of the anastomosis, a 22-F silicon Foley catheter is inserted through the urethra. In the male patient, the two ileoureteral stents (6 F, single J) are inserted via the right lateral port, which is then removed and reinserted alongside the stents, so that the stents do not occupy the port itself after their insertion. In the female patient, the stents can be inserted via the external urethral meatus alongside the Foley catheter. Both stents are delivered into the Studer limb and retrieved into the peritoneal cavity through two separate ileotomy incisions at the proposed site of ureteroneovesical anastomosis. The anterior wall of the pouch is folded over and closed to achieve final configuration. Before completing closure of the pouch, the two ureteral stents and a 12-F cystostomy tube are passed through the wall of the pouch where it is covered by some meso-ileum.

Ureteroneovesical anastomosis is performed in an open side-to-end fashion using two separate 3-0 Vicryl sutures on a RB-1 needle, with one suture each for the anterior and the posterior walls of the spatulated ureteral end. Before completion of anastomosis, a single J-stent is passed into each ureter up to the renal pelvis. The constructed neobladder is irrigated through the Foley catheter and/or cystostomy and any leakage site is repaired by a figure-of-8 stitch.

Surgical Outcomes and Complications

Most of the recent publications on LRC reported the institutions' initial experience regarding technical feasibility and perioperative outcomes (Table 1). In 2004, Hrouda et al. [11] reviewed available data for a total of 54 patients in eight articles regarding LRC. However, the small number of patients and the short duration of follow-up (maximum of 2 years) do not permit any conclusions about its oncologic outcome. We summarize currently available data of oncologic outcomes of LRC for bladder cancer in Table 2. An acceptability of the laparoscopic approach for bladder malignancy remains to proven for long-term oncologic outcomes. Although oncologic data following LRC is limited, Gupta et al. described good outcomes of a 2-year follow-up of their initial experiences of 11 patients undergoing LRC [12]. One patient (9%) had a positive surgical margin and underwent cisplatinum-based chemotherapy; no recurrence was found in their follow-up period. At a mean of 18.4 months' follow-up, all 11 patients had normal renal function and preserved upper tracts, with no evidence of metastasis and no local recurrence.

Recent emphasis on extended pelvic lymphadenectomy for bladder cancer supports such discussion [10]. In 2004, Finelli and colleagues reported their analysis of 22 cases of laparoscopic pelvic lymphadenectomy for bladder cancer from the Cleveland Clinic [10]. The initial 11 patients undergoing a limited dissection were compared with the subsequent 11 consecutive patients undergoing an extended lymphadenectomy. Bilateral extended lymphadenectomy required approximately 1.5 h, while 30–45 min were required for the limited template. Importantly, with a limited lymphadenectomy, the median and mean number of lymph nodes retrieved was 3 and 6 (range 1–15) versus 21 and 18 (range 6–30) for the extended template ($P = 0.001$). The median nodal yield of the laparoscopic extended pelvic lymphadenectomy was in keeping with open surgical series, recommending that at least 10–15 lymph nodes be removed. In the 11 patients with laparoscopic lymphadenectomy, neither port-site dissemination nor local recurrence was found over the short follow-up of 11 months (range 2–43 months).

Laparoscopic radical cystectomy is indeed a complex procedure and requires technically advanced laparoscopic skill. Therefore, a critical appraisal of the attendant complications is essential. In 2003, Sharp and colleagues reported in detail the complications regarding their initial experience of 21 LRCs [14]. All of the 21 were intracorporeally created urinary diversion carried out in the Cleveland Clinic; six major (29%) and nine minor (45%) complications were reported. The major complications included small bowel obstruction (three), and one each of ureteroileal anastomotic leak, urethrovaginal fistula, and bowel perforation with delayed death, while minor complications were mainly related to

TABLE 1. World experience with laparoscopic radical cystectomy and urinary diversion

Technique	Lead author [Ref.]	Institution/location	*n*	Comment on abstract/manuscript or technique
Purely laparoscopic	Gill [1,2,11,14]	Cleveland, USA	30	Purely laparoscopic reconstruction of the urinary diversion
	Türk [9]	Massachusetts, USA and Berlin, Germany	15	Mainz II continent sigmoid-rectal pouch
Laparoscopic-assisted	Van Velthoven [19]	Brussels, Belgium	22	Extracorporeal reconstruction, variety of diversions
	Basillote [16]	Irvine, USA	13	Comparison between LC and open radical cystectomy, extracorporeal reconstruction
	Hemal [15]	New Delhi, India	11	Emphasis on complications of the initial experience with LC. Extracorporeal ileal conduit
	Simonato [20]	Milan, Italy	10	Detailed steps of LC with illustrations. A variety of diversions including intracorporeal and extracorporeal reconstruction
	Denewer [21]	Mnsoura, Egypt	10	Salvage cystectomy after radical radiotherapy. A modified ureterosigmoidostomy diversion through a minilaparotomy (8 cm)
	Abdel-Hakim [22]	Cairo, Egypt	9	Extracorporeal reconstruction of ileal neobladder
	Castillo [19]	Santiago, Chile	7	Extracorporeal reconstruction, Studer neobladder
	Paz [19]	Ashkelon, Israel	7	Comparison between LC and open radical cystectomy, extracorporeal reconstruction
	Popken [19]	Berlin, Germany	7	Extra/intracorporeal reconstruction with a variety of diversions
	Puppo [23]	Pietra Ligure, Italy	5	First transvaginal and laparoscopic approach for bladder cancer. Ileal conduit was accomplished through a minilaparotomy at the stoma site
	Xiao [19]	Guangzhou, China	5	Extracorporeal reconstruction, Indiana pouch

	Huan [19]	Chi Mei, Taiwan	4	Extracorporeal reconstruction, Indiana pouch
	Sung [19]	Pusan, Korea	4	Extracorporeal ileal conduit
	Guazzoni [24]	Milan, Italy	3	Nerve sparing LC with extracorporeal W-shaped neobladder
	Pedraza [19]	New York, USA	2	Patients underwent LC with total ureterectomy and creation of pyelocutaneous ileal conduit was intracorporeally
Hand-assisted	Taylor [25]	Dallas, USA	5	Comparison between hand-assisted cystectomy (5 bladder cancer and 3 benign disease) and open cystectomy with ileal conduit
	McGinnis [26]	Bryn Mawr, USA	7	Hand-assisted LC with extracorporeal ileal conduit
	Fan [19]	Chi Mei, Taiwan	6	Hand-assisted laparoscopic bilateral nephroureterectomy with radical cystectomy (end-stage renal disease)
	Peterson [27]	Tacoma, USA	1	First reported case of hand-assisted LC with extracorporeal ileal conduit
Robotic-assisted	Menon [28]	Detroit, USA	14	Nerve sparing robotic-assisted LC
	Balaji [29]	Omaha, USA	3	LC with robotic assistance for intracorporeal suturing of the ureter-ileal conduit anastomosis (2 patients with interstitial cystitis)
	Beecken [30]	Frankfurt, Germany	1	First reported case of robotic-assisted LC with intracorporeal orthotopic neobladder
Other	Goharderakhshan [14]	Harbor City, USA	25	Series focusing on complications associated with LC. Reconstructive technique not detailed
	Vallancien [14]	Paris, France	20	Prostate sparing cystectomy. Reconstructive technique not detailed

Adapted from the Table 1 in Ukimura O, Moinzadeh A, Gill IS. (2005) Laparoscopic radical cystectomy and urinary diversion. Current Urology Reports: in press.

Table 2. Oncological outcomes

Lead author (year) [Ref.]	N	Technique (reconstruction)	Margins	Lymphadenectomy (n node, range)	Mean (range) months at stated follow-up	Overall survival (n)
Puppo (1995) [23]	5	Lap (extra)	Not stated	Limited (not stated)	10.8 (6–18)	5
Denewer (1999) [21]	10	Lap (extra)	Not stated	Limited (not stated)	Not stated	9
Turk (2001) [9]	5	Lap (purely intra)	5/5 negative	Limited (not stated)	Not stated	5
Abdel-Hakim (2002) [22]	9	Lap (extra)	9/9 negative	Limited (n = 2–4)	Not stated	9
Simonato (2003) [20]	10	Lap (extra)	10/10 negative	Limited (not stated)	12.3 (5–18)	10
Menon (2003) [28]	17	Robot (extra)	17/17 negative	Limited (n = 4–27)	Not stated (2–11)	17
Hemal (2004) [15]	11	Lap (extra)	10/11 negative	Limited (not stated)	18.4 (1–48)	10
Basillotte (2004) [16]	13	Lap (extra)	12/13 negative	Limited (not stated)	Not stated	13
Taylor (2004) [25]	5	HAL (extra)	4/5 negative	(Extended not stated)	Not stated	5
Gill (2004) [10]	22	Lap (purely intra)	21/22 negative	11/22 Extended (n = 21, 6–30)	11 (2–43)	18

Adapted from Table 2 in Ukimura O, Moinzadeh A, Gill IS (2005) Laparoscopic radical cystectomy and urinary diversion. Current Urology Reports: in press.

Lap, laparoscopy; HAL, hand-assisted laparoscopy.

prolonged ileus. Table 3 is a comparison of technique characteristics between intracorporeal and extracorporeal LRC.

In 2004, Hemal et al. reported their initial experiences of 11 patients who underwent LRC and an open-hand sewn ileal conduit [15]. One case (9%) had a positive margin and five (45%) had procedure-specific complications. Three intraoperative complications were found including injury to the external iliac vein in one patient and a small rectal tear in two, all repaired by laparoscopic freehand suturing. Additional laparoscopic-related complications were subcutaneous emphysema and hypercarbia in one patient, necessitating conversion to open surgery. The authors described that LRC is associated with complications similar to those seen with other laparoscopic and open surgery procedures, especially during the initial period [15]. In Table 4 we review complications of LRC described in the previous studies having 10 or more patients.

Recently, Basillote et al. retrospectively compared perioperative outcomes of radical cystectomy with ileal neobladder between 11 men who underwent open approach and 13 men who underwent the laparoscopic-assisted approach [16]. They suggested that the laparoscopic approach provided a significant decrease in postoperative pain (parenteral morphine-equivalent use: open, 144 vs laparoscopy, 61; $P = 0.04$) and quicker recovery [(i) start of oral liquids: open, 5 vs laparoscopy, 2.8, $P = 0.004$; (ii) start of oral solids: open, 6.1 vs laparoscopy, 4.1, $P = 0.002$; (iii) hospital stay: open, 8.4 vs laparoscopy, 5.1, $P = 0.0004$; (iv) light work resumed: open, 19 vs laparoscopy, 11, $P = 0.0001$) without a significant increase in operative time and with similar complication rates. The authors concluded that the laparoscopic-assisted approach contributes to decreased postoperative pain and quicker recovery, with similar complication rates to the open approach [16]. Table 5 is a summary of surgical outcomes of LRC in the major reports.

Future Directions

An increasing number of major medical institutions have performed LRC. However, the most challenging aspect is the laparoscopic reconstructive urinary diversion. Although there is considerable difference of opinion and clinical practice regarding urinary diversion as well as bladder substitution, currently, orthotopic ileal neobladders represent the most physiological bladder substitute after radical cystectomy for bladder cancer, and have been used in both male and female patients. However, considerable disadvantages of using intestinal segments in urinary tract reconstruction have been reported, including metabolic complications, complicated infections, stone and tumor formation, and a variety of surgical risks associated with bowel surgery. These disturbances are exaggerated in patients with compromised renal function as well as in children. As such, the search for the ideal urinary bladder substitute continues. In the near future, novel bladder substitution methods such as tissue engineering [17] and ureteral augmentation [18] or the use of absorbable endoscopic staples may

TABLE 3. Comparing technique characteristics between intracorporeal versus extracorporeal

	Intracorporeal reconstruction		Extracorporeal reconstruction		
Lead author	Gill [1,2,11,14]	Turk [9]	Van Velthoven [19]	Simonato [20]	Basillote [16]
n	22	5	22	10	13
Urinary diversion, *n*	Ileal conduit, 14 (intracorporeal) Orthotopic, 6 (intracorporeal) Indiana pouch, 2 (extra)	Rectal sigmoid pouch, all 5 purely intracorporeal	Orthotopic, 11 ileal conduit, 6 Mainz II, 2 Kock pouch, 2	Orthotopic, 6 Sigmoid uret., 2 Cutaneous uret., 2	Orthotopic, all 13
Skin incision	6 port site only for ileal conduit and orthotopic (20 mm extension of umbilical port incision for Indiana)	6 port site only	5 port plus additional skin incision	5 port and 50 mm midline skin incision above umbilicus	5 port and low abdominal Pfannenstiel incision (150 mm)
Overall operative time (range), h	8.6	7.4 (6.9–7.9)	7.4	7.1 for orthotopic 5.8 for sigmoid uret. 4.7 for cutaneous uret.	8.0 (8.0 h ± 77 min)
Cystectomy + lymphadenectomy (LA) time	Extended LA ($n = 11$) added 1.5 h	Not stated	Not stated	166 min (150–180) (with limited LA)	Not stated
Blood loss (range), ml	490	245 (190–300)	840 (210–400)	310 (220–440)	1000 (1000 ± 414)
Hospital stay, days	Not stated	10	Not stated	8.1 for orthotopic 8 for sigmoid uret. 5 for Cutaneous uret.	5.1 (5.1 ± 1.2)

Days for oral intake	8	Liquid 3	Not stated	3–6	Liquid 2.8 (2.8 ± 1.4) Solid 4.1 (4.1 ± 1.2)
Complications	6 prolonged ileus 3 bowel obstruction 2 deep venous thrombosis 1 bowel perforation 1 ureteroileal leak 1 urethrovaginal fistula 1 postoperative bleed 1 deep pelvic vein injury	All discharged with no intra- or postop. complication (with continent, normal renal function, mild hyperchlolemic acidosis)	1 rectal injury (other was not detailed)	1 Grade 3 bilateral hydronephrosis 1 Grade 2 bilateral hydronephrosis 1 monolateral hydronephrosis 2 metabolic acidosis	1 ureteral obstruction 1 bladder neck contracture 1 epididymal abscess 1 wound dehiscence 1 obturator nerve paresis 1 pyelonephritis 1 pouchitis
Note for oncological outcomes	21/22 negative margin 6/22 (27%) had positive LN 3/22 died of metastasis	5/5 negative margin	Not stated	10/10 negative margin, 2 had diffusive metastasis after 6 months	12/13 negative margin 1 had prostate cancer with a positive apical margin
Follow-up, months	Mean 11 (range 2–43)	Not stated	Not stated	Mean 12.3 (range 5–18)	Not stated
No. overall survival	18	5	Not stated	10	13

Adapted from the Table 3 in Ukimura O, Moinzadeh A, Gill IS (2005) Laparoscopic radical cystectomy and urinary diversion. Current Urology Reports: in press.

TABLE 4. Complications in studies with complication descriptions (n = 10 or more)

Lead author (year) [Ref.]	n	No. of comlications	Description of complications	Dealing and event
Basillote (2004) [16]	13	8 4 major (31%)	1 ureteral obstruction	Percutaneous nephrostomy
			1 bladder neck contracture	Reoperation
			1 epididymal abscess	Orchiectomy
			1 wound dehiscence	Reoperation
			1 obturator nerve paresis	Physical therapy
			1 pyelonephritis	Intravenous antibiotics
			1 pouchitis	Intravenous antibiotics
			1 positive margin at prostate apex	
Simonato (2003) [20]	10	5	2 metabolic acidosis	Sodium bicarbonate administration
			1 Grade 3 bilateral hydronephrosis	
			1 Grade 2 bilateral hydronephrosis	
			1 Grade 2 monolateral hydronephrosis	
Denewer (1999) [21]	10	6	1 external iliac artery clipped, leading to 1 postoperative deep venous thrombus	Vascular resection anastomosis from open part Thrombolytics
			1 reactionary hemorrhage	Re-exploration and delayed death
			1 urine leak	Conservative drainage
			1 pelvic collection in diabetes patient	Ultrasound guided drainage
			1 pyelonephritis in diabetes patient	Parenteral antibiotics
Menon (2003) [28]	17	15	13 bilharziasis with periureteric, perivesicular, and perivesical scarring	
			1 bleeding	Re-exploration
			1 for a malfunction of lens	Open conversion
Hemal (2004) [15]	11	6 3 major (27%)	2 small rectal tear	Laparoscopic suturing
			1 external iliac vein injury	Laparoscopic suturing
			1 subcutaneous emphysema	Resolved over 4 days
			1 hypercarbia	Open conversion and delayed death
			1 positive margin	Cisplatinum-based chemotherapy
Gill (2004) [10,14]	22	16 6 major (27%)	6 prolonged ileus	Conservative management
			3 bowel obstruction	Open conversion
			2 deep venous thrombosis	Thrombolytics
			1 urethrovaginal fistula	Open conversion
			1 bowel perforation	Open conversion and delayed death
			1 ureteroileal leak	Open conversion
			1 postoperative bleed	Laparoscopic suturing
			1 deep pelvic vein injury	Laparoscopic suturing

Adapted from the Table 4 in Ukimura O, Moinzadeh A, Gill IS (2005) Laparoscopic radical cystectomy and urinary diversion. Current Urology Reports: in press.

Table 5. Operative outcomes

Lead author (year)	Puppo (1995) [23]	Denewer (1999) [21]	Turk (2001) [9]	Abdel-Hakim (2002) [22]	Simonato (2003) [20]	Menon (2003) [28]	Hemal (2004) [15]	Basillotte (2004) [16]	Taylor (2004) [25]	Gill (2004) [11,14]
n	5	10	5	9	10	17	11	13	8	22
Technique (reconstruction)	Transvaginal and lap-assisted (extra)	Lap-assisted (extra)	Purely intracorporeal laparoscopic	Lap-assisted (extra)	Lap-assisted (extra)	Robot-assisted (extra)	Lap-assisted (extra)	Lap-assisted (extra)	Hand-assisted (extra)	Purely intracorporeal laparoscopic
Urinary diversion	Ileal cond., 4 Cutaneous, 1	Sigmoid-pouch, 10 (extra)	Rectal-sigmoid-pouch, 5 (purely intra)	Orthotopic, 9 (extra)	Orthotopic, 6 Sigmoid, 2 Cutaneous, 2 (extra)	Orthotopic, 14 Ileal cond., 3 (extra)	Ileal cond., 11 (extra)	Orthotopic, 13 (extra)	Ileal cond., 8 (extra)	Ileal cond., 14 Orthotopic, 6 (intra) Indiana, 2 (extra)
Mean (range) operative duration (h)	7.2 (6–9)	3.6 (3.3–4.1)	7.4 (6.9–7.9)	8.3 (6.5–12)	Orthotopic, 7.1 Sigmoid, 5.8 Cutaneous, 4.7	Orthotopic, 5.1 Ileal cond., 4.3	6.1 (4.3–8)	8.0 h (±77 min)	6.7 (5.5–7.7)	8.6
Blood loss (ml), *transfusion	*3 pts transfused 2–6 units	*Transfused mean 2.2 unit, range 2–3	245 (190–300)	150–500	310 (220–440)	<150	530 (300–900)	1000 ± 414	637 (400–1000), *transfused in 2 pts	490
Ileus (days)	2.6 (2–4)	Not stated	Not stated	Not stated	3.3 (1–5)	Not stated	Not stated	Not stated	1 prolonged	6 prolonged ileus 3 bowel obstruction
Length of stay (days)	10.6 (7–18)	10–13	10 (in all 5)	Not stated	Orthotopic, 8.1 Sigmoid, 8 Cutaneous, 5	Nor stated	10.5	5.1 ± 1.2	6.4 (3–10)	Not stated
Time to oral intake (days)	2–4	Not stated	Liquid 3	3	3–6	Not stated	Not stated	Liquid 2.8 Solid 4.1	4.5 (3–8)	8
Time to return to work (days)	Not stated	Not stated	Not stated	Not stated	Not stated	Not stated	26	11.0 ± 1.9	21–28	Not stated
Follow-up months	11 (6–16)	Not stated	Not stated	Not stated	12.3 (5–18)	Not stated	18.4 (1–48)	Not stated	Not stated	11 (2–43)
Functional outcomes	4/5 discharged with no postop. complications, 1 discharged after 18 days due to obesity and diabetic problems	All continence, 1 uretero-sigmoid urine leak, 1 pyelo-nephritis	All 5 with continent and no obstruction of upper urinary tract in urogram on 10th postop. day	No complications in pouchgram on 10th post-op. day	2 bilateral hydronephrosis and metabolic acidosis, 1 monolateral hydronephrosis	13 bilharziasis with peri-ureteric, peri-vesicular, and perivesical scarring	All had normal renal function and preserved upper urinary tracts	1 ureteral obstruction 1 bladder neck contracture 1 obturator nerve paresis	1 upper gastrointestinal bleed 1 rectal injury and ileus	1 ureteroileal leak 1 urethro-vaginal fistula

Adapted from Table 5 in Ukimura O, Moinzadeh A, Gill IS (2005) Laparoscopic radical cystectomy and urinary diversion. Current Urology Reports: in press.
cond., conduct; lap, laparoscopy; pts, patients.

decrease the technical difficulty associated with laparoscopic reconstructive urinary diversion.

Conclusions

As reports of recent growing experience are published from major medical centers throughout the world, minimally invasive surgery for bladder cancer and urinary diversion reconstruction is gaining acceptance. Prospective assessments of oncologic and functional outcomes are awaited to define whether laparoscopic radical cystectomy and urinary diversion reconstruction is a viable alternative to the standard open surgical approach.

References

1. Gill IS, Fergany A, Klein EA, Kaouk JH, Sung GT, Meraney AM, Savage SJ, Ulchaker JC, Novick AC (2000) Laparoscopic radical cystoprostatectomy with ileal conduit performed completely intracorporeally: the initial 2 cases. Urology 56:26–29
2. Gill IS, Kaouk JH, Meraney AM, Desai MM, Ulchaker JC, Klein EA, Savage SJ, Sung GT (2002) Laparoscopic radical cystectomy and continent orthotopic ileal neobladder performed completely intracorporeally: the initial experience. J Urol 168:13–18
3. Parra RO, Andrus CH, Jones JP, Boullier JA (1992) Laparoscopic cystectomy: initial report on a new treatment for the retained bladder. J Urol 148:1140–1144
4. Sanchez de Badajoz E, Gallego Perales JL, Reche Rosado A, Gutierrez de la Cruz JM, Jimenez Garrido A (1995) Laparoscopic cystectomy and ileal conduit: case report. J Endourol 9:59–62
5. Kozminski M, Partamian KO (1992) Case report of laparoscopic ileal loop conduit. J Endourol 6:147–150
6. Anderson KR, Fadden PT, Kerbl K, McDougall EM, Clayman RV (1995) Laparoscopic assisted continent urinary diversion in the pig. J Urol 154:1934–1938
7. Fergany AF, Gill IS, Kaouk JH, Meraney AM, Hafez KS, Sung GT (2001) Laparoscopic intracorporeally constructed ileal conduit after porcine cystoprostatectomy. J Urol 166:285–288
8. Kaouk JH, Gill IS, Desai MM, Meraney AM, Fergany AF, Abdelsamea A, Carvalhal EF, Skacel M, Sung GT (2001) Laparoscopic orthotopic ileal neobladder. J Endourol 15:131–142
9. Turk I, Deger S, Winkelmann B, Schonberger B, Loening SA (2001) Laparoscopic radical cystectomy with continent urinary diversion (rectal sigmoid pouch) performed completely intracorporeally: the initial 5 cases. J Urol 165:1863–1866
10. Finelli A, Gill IS, Desai MM, Moinzadeh A, Magi-Galluzzi C, Kaouk JH (2004) Laparoscopic extended pelvic lymphadenectomy for bladder cancer: Technique and initial outcomes. J Urol 172:1809–1812
11. Hrouda D, Adeyoju AA, Gill IS (2004) Laparoscopic radical cystectomy and urinary diversion: fad or future? BJU Int 94:501–505
12. Gupta NP, Gill IS, Fergany A, Nabi G (2002) Laparoscopic radical cystectomy with intracorporeal ileal conduit diversion: five cases with a 2-year follow-up. BJU Int 90:391–396

13. Stein JP, Cai J, Groshen S, Skinner DG (2003) Risk factors for patients with pelvic lymph node metastases following radical cystectomy with en bloc pelvic lymphadenectomy: concept of lymph node density. J Urol 170:35–41
14. AUA (2003) Abstracts: American Urological Association Annual Meeting, April 26–May 1, 2003, Chicago, Illinois. p 169 Supplement
15. Hemal AK, Kumar R, Seth A, Gupta NP (2004) Complications of laparoscopic radical cystectomy during the initial experience. Int J Urol 11:483–488
16. Basillote JB, Abdelshehid C, Ahlering TE, Shanberg AM (2004) Laparoscopic assisted radical cystectomy with ileal neobladder: a comparison with the open approach. J Urol 172:489–493
17. Atala A (2004) Tissue engineering for the replacement of organ function in the genitourinary system. Am J Transplant 4 Suppl 6:58–73
18. Desai MM, Gill IS, Goel M, Abreu SC, Ramani AP, Bedaiwy MA, Kaouk JH, Matin SF, Steinberg AP, Brainard J, Robertson D, Sung GT (2003) Ureteral tissue balloon expansion for laparoscopic bladder augmentation: survival study. J Endourol 17:283–293
19. Anonymous (2003) Abstracts: 21st World Congress on Endourology and SWL, September 21–24. J Endourol 17 Suppl 1:A80
20. Simonato A, Gregori A, Lissiani A, Bozzola A, Galli S, Gaboardi F (2003) Laparoscopic radical cystoprostatectomy: a technique illustrated step by step. Eur Urol 44:132–138
21. Denewer A, Kotb S, Hussein O, El-Maadawy M (1999) Laparoscopic assisted cystectomy and lymphadenectomy for bladder cancer: initial experience. World J Surg 23:608–611
22. Abdel-Hakim AM, Bassiouny F, Abdel Azim MS, Rady I, Mohey T, Habib I, Fathi H (2002) Laparoscopic radical cystectomy with orthotopic neobladder. J Endourol 16: 377–381
23. Puppo P, Perachino M, Ricciotti G, Bozzo W, Gallucci M, Carmignani G (1995) Laparoscopically assisted transvaginal radical cystectomy. Eur Urol 27:80–84
24. Guazzoni G, Cestari A, Colombo R, Lazzeri M, Montorsi F, Nava L, Losa A, Rigatti P (2003) Laparoscopic nerve- and seminal-sparing cystectomy with orthotopic ileal neobladder: the first three cases. Eur Urol 44:567–572
25. Taylor GD, Duchene DA, Koeneman KS (2004) Hand assisted laparoscopic cystectomy with minilaparotomy ileal conduit: series report and comparison with open cystectomy. J Urol 172:1291–1296
26. McGinnis DE, Hubosky SG, Bergmann LS (2004) Hand-assisted laparoscopic cystoprostatectomy and urinary diversion. J Endourol 18:383–386
27. Peterson AC, Lance RS, Ahuja S (2002) Laparoscopic hand assisted radical cystectomy with ileal conduit urinary diversion. J Urol 168:2103–2105
28. Menon M, Hemal AK, Tewari A, Shrivastava A, Shoma AM, El-Tabey NA, Shaaban A, Abol-Enein H, Ghoneim MA (2003) Nerve-sparing robot-assisted radical cystoprostatectomy and urinary diversion. BJU Int 92:232–236
29. Balaji KC, Yohannes P, McBride CL, Oleynikov D, Hemstreet GP 3rd (2004) Feasibility of robot-assisted totally intracorporeal laparoscopic ileal conduit urinary diversion: initial results of a single institutional pilot study. Urology 63:51–55
30. Beecken WD, Wolfram M, Engl T, Bentas W, Probst M, Blaheta R, Oertl A, Jonas D, Binder J (2003) Robotic-assisted laparoscopic radical cystectomy and intra-abdominal formation of an orthotopic ileal neobladder. Eur Urol 44:337–339

Robot-Assisted Radical Cystectomy and Urinary Diversion in Bladder Cancer

Ashok K. Hemal and Mani Menon

Summary. The potential advantages of robot-assisted surgery can be utilized in complex and advanced uro-oncologic surgery. The technique of robot-assisted radical cystectomy (RRC) for patients with bladder cancer in males and females was developed based on principles of open and laparoscopic surgery with modifications using the daVinci system. This procedure employs precise and rapid radical cystectomy with minimal blood loss. Urinary diversions such as orthotopic neobladder or ileal conduit can be performed totally intracorporeally, or the bowel segment is exteriorized from the incision used to deliver the specimen and the orthotopic neobladder or ileal conduit is reconstructed. At this point in time, performing urinary diversion extracorporeally reduces operative time in comparison to performing the procedure totally intracorporeally.

Keywords. Robot-assisted cystectomy, Urinary diversion, Bladder cancer, Uro-oncologic surgery

Introduction

Carcinoma of the urinary bladder is the most common malignancy of the urinary tract and almost 25% of cases with newly diagnosed bladder cancer have muscle-invasive disease [1]. Radical cystectomy is the most effective mode of treatment for these patients. Open surgery has been the standard option for these patients but is associated with complications in up to 30% of cases [2–4]. Among the various methods of urinary diversion, ileal conduit is a standard and versatile option against which newer techniques including orthotopic neobladders can be compared. On the other hand, the high complication rates associated with urinary diversion into the rectum makes this option less desirable in a patient with a significant life expectancy [5].

Vattikuti Urology Institute, Henry Ford Hospital, 2799 West Grand Boulevard, Detroit, MI 48202, USA

Refinements in surgical technique with respect to continent orthotopic diversion, as well as the incorporation of nerve sparing for preservation of sexual function, have allowed not only effective cancer control but also significant improvements in the quality of life [6]. These advances in surgical technique and improved instrumentation have allowed complex surgeries such as radical prostatectomy to be performed laparoscopically and with more versatility and excellent outcome using robots [7,8]. Laparoscopic radical cystectomy has been well described in the literature with reconstruction of intracorporeal and extracorporeal urinary diversions (Tables 1 and 2) [9–16].

Basillote et al. recently reported their cystectomy experience, comparing open surgery with laparoscopic assistance and creation of an ileal neobladder [17]. They found that patients experienced decreased postoperative pain and quicker recovery without a significant increase in operative time and intracorporeal urinary diversion, proving the possibility that it can be done purely laparoscopically [17]. However, despite the feasibility, the use of laparoscopy for cystectomy has been limited to very few centers across the world due to potential complications and a steep learning curve [18]. The experience gained from robot-assisted laparoscopic radical prostatectomy by our team was used as an interface to develop the technique of robot-assisted radical cystectomy, based on anatomic delineation with incorporation of principles of open radical cystectomy. At the

Table 1. Laparoscopic radical cystectomy (LRC) and ileal conduit (IC) urinary diversion

	Puppo et al. [9]	Hemal et al. [10]	Gill et al. [11]	Gupta et al. [12]
No. of cases	5	9	2	5
Procedure	Lap.-assisted transvaginal RC + IC	LRC + IC	LRC + IC	LRC + IC
Urinary diversion (intra/extracorporeal)	Extracorporeal	Extracorporeal	Intracorporeal	Intracorporeal
Operation time, h (range)	7.2 (6–9)	6.48 (5–8.1)	10.8 (10–11.5)	7.5 (7–8)
Blood loss (ml)/transfusion	3 transfused 2–6 units	533.3 ml (300–800)	1100 (1000–1200)	360 (300–400)/nil transfused
Length of stay (days)	10.6 (8–18)	10.88 (8–21)	6	7 (6–22)
Time to oral intake (days)	2–4	NS	4	3
Time to return to work (days)	NS	26.44	NS	20 (13–35)
Follow-up (months)	10.8	19	NS	24
Complications	None	3 minor, 4 major[a]	None	[b]

NS, not stated.

[a] Minor: subcutaneous emphysema, Subacute intestinal obstruction (SAIO), deep vein thrombosis; major: rectal tear (2), external iliac vein tear, hypercarbia.

[b] One small bowel obstruction, one self-limiting abdominal distension.

TABLE 2. Laparoscopic radical cystectomy (LRC) and continent diversion—orthotopic ileal neobladder (OIN)

	Gaboardi et al. [13]	Gill et al. [14]	Simonato et al. [15]	Abdel-Hakim et al. [16]
No. of cases	1	2	6	8
Procedure	LRC + OIN	LRC + OIN	LRC + OIN	LRC + OIN
Intra/extracorporeal	Intra + extra	Intracorporeal	Extracorporeal	Extracorporeal
Operation time, h (range)	7.5	9.5 (8.5–10.5)	7.1	8.3 (6.5–12)
Blood loss (ml)	350	300 (200–400)	310 (220–440)	150–500
Length of stay (days)	7	8.5 (5–12)	8.1 (7–9)	NS
Time to oral intake (days)	2	2–4	3–5	3
Follow-up (months)		1–13	9.3 (5–15)	NS
Complications	None	[a]	None	None

[a] Bleeding duodenal ulcer.

time of writing our team has modest experience of 30 cases of robotic-assisted radical cystectomy procedures.

Surgical Technique

Patient Preparation and Port Placement

The patient presents on the morning of surgery after undergoing a formal bowel preparation. After the induction of general anesthesia, all upper extremity pressure points are padded and the patient is positioned in the extended lithotomy position.

The nuances of port placement have been recently described in detail [19]. In brief, to achieve transperitoneal access, pneumoperitoneum is created using a Veress needle in the supraumbilical region (Ethicon Endosurgery, Albuquerque, NM, USA). Upon insufflation to 15 mmHg, a 12-mm primary port is inserted and the peritoneal cavity is inspected with a 30° laparoscope. Two 8-mm robotic instrument ports are placed at the lateral edge of the rectus muscle at a point 2 cm below the umbilicus on each respective side. A second 12-mm port is placed in the right iliac fossa approximately 3 cm above the iliac crest. A 5-mm port is placed between the robotic and 12-mm port on right side and another 5-mm port is placed on the left side 3 cm above the iliac crest. The daVinci robot is then docked over the patient.

Dissection in Recto-Vesical Pouch

The laparoscope is positioned on the daVinci robot with the 30° lens angled downward. An inverted U-shaped incision is made in the peritoneum of the cul-de-sac and extended to a point 2 cm proximal to the bifurcation of the common iliac artery. Dissection is started at the point where the ureters cross the iliac vessels, and follows the course of the ureters proximally and distally after identifying the vas deferens, the dissection can be extended proximally. The ureters, located on the under-surface of the posterior peritoneum, are dissected above the bifurcation of the iliac vessels proximally, and to the ureteral-vesical junction (UVJ) distally.

The ureter is then clipped and divided. Sometimes, the inferior vesical pedicles may be identified, which are clipped and divided The posterior layer of Denonvilliers' fascia is then incised in the midline and the plane between the rectum and the prostate is developed inferiorly. If nerve-sparing radical cystoprostatectomy is performed, then dissection is limited to a plane between the seminal vesicle and the posterior layer of Denonvilliers' fascia. The rectoprostatic plane is now developed by dividing Denonvilliers' fascia. Finally, the bladder is dropped by incising lateral to the medial umbilical ligament. The incision then curves medially under the rectus abdominis, transecting the medial umbilical ligaments and the urachus.

Mobilization of Bladder, Dissection of the Prostate, and Preservation of the Neurovascular Bundles

For control of the bladder pedicles and dorsal vein complex, the superior vesical pedicle is clipped and divided at its origin. The anterior trunk of the internal iliac artery continues as the inferior vesical artery, which gives off vesical branches, is secured if not done earlier. The endopelvic fascia is opened lateral to the prostate and the dorsal vein complex is ligated. The apex of the urethra is freed from the rectourethralis bluntly or with scissors. We use the seminal vesicles as an operative landmark to avoid injury to the neurovascular bundles where the dissection occurs in a plane between the posterior surface of seminal vesicle and the posterior layer of Denonvilliers' fascia. The dissection is performed with daVinci articulated scissors and bipolar forceps. The neurovascular bundle is reflected laterally, leaving a layer of Denonvilliers' fascia on the surface of the rectum [20].

Division of Urethra and Removal of Specimen

With careful dissection the urethra is mobilized and divided close to the apex of prostate using articulated robotic scissors, with the goal of preserving as much length as possible. The posterior striated sphincter should be divided carefully. The specimen is entrapped in a laparoscopic Endocatch II bag (US Surgical, Norwalk, CT, USA). At this point the daVinci system is removed and the specimen is retrieved through a 5–6-cm incision placed midway between the umbilicus and pubic symphysis. Through the same incision, a segment of ileum is extracted, isolated, detubularized, and reconfigured extracorporeally. Through the bladder extraction incision it is possible to perform the following diversions: (1) ileal conduit, (2) W-pouch with a serosal-lined tunnel, sigmoid neobladder and (3) double chimney or T-pouch with a serosal-lined tunnel. The techniques of ileal conduit reconstruction and orthotopic substitution are described in previous reports [6,21–24]. The pouch, which was created extracorporeally, is then placed in the pelvis and a Foley catheter passed through the urethra and into the pouch. The abdominal incision is closed and the daVinci system is redocked. The urethroneovesicostomy is performed robotically using a double-armed 3–0 Polydioxanone suture in a continuous fashion, as previously described [6].

Extended Pelvic Lymphadenectomy

If lymphadenectomy is not performed at the beginning then it is performed after completion of the cystectomy portion of the operation. Using the 0° lens, the robotic bipolar cautery, and the robotic scissors, nodal tissue is cautiously cleared. The limits of the dissection are from the genitofemoral nerve laterally, the bifurcation of the common iliac artery proximally, and the node of Cloquet distally. Care is taken to preserve the obturator nerve.

Comments

Reports on laparoscopic radical cystectomy (LRC) have been published by several authors. Parra et al. [25] performed the first laparoscopic simple cystectomy for infection in a retained bladder, but the first case of radical cystectomy with extracorporeal construction of an ileal conduit was reported by Sanchez de Badajoz et al. [26]. Since then many authors have reported performing LRC with extracorporeal urinary diversion from the site of specimen removal or by a minilaparotomy incision. To date since 1992, fewer than 500 reports exist in the world literature. Gill et al. were the first to report two cases of LRC and intracorporeal ileal conduit formation [11]. Turk et al. were the first to report five cases of LRC and intracorporeal continent (rectosigmoid pouch) urinary diversion and transrectal specimen retrieval [27]. Gill et al. also performed LRC and an orthotopic neobladder (Studer) in two patients [14]. This is the first report in the literature where authors have described the technique and demonstrated the feasibility of laparoscopic radical cystectomy and creation of a continent orthotopic ileal neobladder. Hemal et al. reviewed the complications of laparoscopic radical cystectomy in their initial experience in order to reduce their occurrence and allow development of a better technique [18].

Despite the feasibility of LRC, the skill required to perform such an operation remains solely in the hands of highly experienced laparoscopic surgeons. Intraoperative blood loss and subsequent need for transfusion have always been associated with radical pelvic surgery such as prostatectomy and cystectomy. One of the most notable advantages of LRC is the decreased blood loss and low transfusion rates as compared to open surgery. However, the procedure is difficult to learn and restricted to those well versed in complex laparoscopic surgery. We sought to develop a technique for robot-assisted radical cystectomy (RARC) that would combine the minimally invasive advantages of laparoscopy with the technical advantages of robotics, as has been demonstrated in robot-assisted radical prostatectomy. To date only a few reported small series exist and these are shown in Table 3. Robotic assistance also allows identification and preservation of the neurovascular bundles with unprecedented precision [6,20]. In addition, this approach offers other advantages such as three-dimensional visualization, greater degrees of freedom, lack of tremor, and the intuitiveness of surgical motion. These enhancements are especially highlighted during reconstruction phases of pelvic surgery as in creation of the urethra-neovesicostomy. As a result, we feel that these features increase surgical precision and reduce surgeon fatigue, especially when performing difficult pelvis surgery such as radical cystectomy.

A potential disadvantage of this technology often cited is the lack of tactile sensation. The need for tactile feedback, however, makes sense in the setting of performing open pelvic surgery, which is often deep, surrounded by neurovascular structures, and obstructed by anatomy such as the bony pelvis. In laparoscopic surgery, especially with robotic assistance, we have found that the lack of tactile feedback was compensated for by the improvement in depth perception from three-dimensional visualization with 10× magnification.

TABLE 3. Published literature on robotic radical cystectomy

Authors	Menon et al. [21]	Beecken et al.[23]	Menon et al. [22]	Yohannes et al. [24]
No. of cases	14 Men	1	3	2
Technique of port (#) placement	5–6 ports	Minilaparotomy, 5 ports	5–6 ports	5 ports
Lymphadenectomy	B/L EPLND	B/L PLND	B/L EPLND	B/L PLND
Operation time (min)	RRC: 140 UD: 120 (IC), 168 (ONB)	RRC + UD: 510	RRC: 150, 160, 170 UD: 130, 190, 170	10 and 12 h
Blood loss (cc)	<150	200	150, 250, 100	435, 1800
Surgical margins	Free of tumor infiltration	Negative	Negative	In 1 case perivesical invasion
Urinary diversion	Ileal conduit: 2	UD: Hautmann ileal neobladder	Ileal conduit: 1	In both cases ileal conduit was reconstructed
	W-Pouch neobladder: 9	Midline incision was extended to exteriorized ileum for ileo-ileal anastomosis	W-Pouch neobladder: 1	
	Double chimney: 2 T Pouch: 1		T Pouch: 1	

B/L EPLND, bilateral extended pelvic lymphadenectomy; IC, ileal conduit; ONB, orthotopic neobladder; RRC, robotic radical cystectomy; UD, urinary diversion.

Conclusions

Although minimally invasive approaches to urologic cancers such as muscle invasive urothelial carcinoma are in their infancy, robotic assistance confers many advantages in performing a difficult operation even in experienced hands. Increased use and refinements in surgical technique may serve to increase the use of robotic assistance in treating bladder cancer. Our institution has certainly seen this in treating prostate cancer. If oncologic outcomes are shown to be equivocal on long-term follow-up, at the very minimum better visualization and use of robotic technology, coupled with minimal blood loss and less morbidity, may contribute to the increasing use of robotic assistance in the future.

References

1. Messing EM, Young TB, Hunt VB, Gilchrist KW, Newtonma, Brammll, Higgen WJ, Greenberg EB, Kuglitsch ME, Wegnke JD (1995) Comparison of bladder cancer outcome in men undergoing hematuria home screening versus those with standard clinical presentations. Urology 45:387–396
2. Cookson MS, Chang SS, Wells N, Parekh DJ, Smith JA Jr (2003) Complications of radical cystectomy for nonmuscle invasive disease: Comparison with muscle invasive disease. J Urol 169:101–104
3. Stein JP, Lieskovsky G, Cote R, Groshen S, Feng AC, Boyds, Skirnez E, Bochner B, Thangathurai D, Mikhail M, Raghvan D, Skinner DG (2001) Radical cystectomy in the treatment of invasive bladder cancer: long-term results in 1,054 patients. J Clin Oncol 19:666–675
4. Figueroa AJ, Stein JP, Dickinson M, Skinner EC, Thangathurai D, Mikhail MS, Boyd SD, Leiskovsdy G, Skinner DG (1998) Radical cystectomy for elderly patients with bladder carcinoma: an updated experience with 404 patients. Cancer 83:141–147
5. Messing EM, Catalona W (1998) Urothelial tumors of the urinary tract. In: Walsh PC, Retik AB, Vaughan ED Jr, Wein AJ (eds) Campbell's urology, 7th edn. Saunders, Philadelphia, pp 2327–2411
6. Hemal AK, Abol-Enein H, Tewari A, Shrivastava A, Shoma AM, Ghoneim MA, Menon M (2004) Robotic radical cystectomy and urinary diversion in the management of bladder cancer. Urol Clin North Am 31(4):719–729
7. Menon M, Hemal AK, Team VIP (2004) Vattikuti Institute prostatectomy: a technique of robotic radical prostatectomy: experience in more than 1000 cases. J Endourol 18(7):611–619
8. Menon M, Tewari A, Peabody JO, Shrivastava A, Kaul S, Bhandari A, Hemal AK (2004) Vattikuti Institute prostatectomy, a technique of robotic radical prostatectomy for management of localized carcinoma of the prostate: experience of over 1100 cases. Urol Clin North Am 31(4):701–717
9. Puppo P, Perachino M, Ricciotti G, Bozzo W, Gallucci M, Carmignani G (1995) Laparoscopically assisted transvaginal radical cystectomy. Eur Urol 27:80–84
10. Hemal AK, Singh I, Kumar R (2003) Laparoscopic radical cystectomy and ileal conduit reconstruction: preliminary experience. J Endourol 17(10):911–916

11. Gill IS, Fergany A, Klein AE, Kaouk JH, Sung GT, Merarey AM, Savage SJ, Ulchaker JC, Novick AC (2000) Laparoscopic radical cystoprostatectomy with ileal conduit performed completely intracorporeally: the initial 2 cases. Urology 56:26–29
12. Gupta NP, Gill IS, Fergany A, Nabi G (2002) Laparoscopic radical cystectomy with intracorporeal ileal conduit diversion: five cases with a 2 year follow-up. BJU Int 90:391–396
13. Gaboardi F, Simonato A, Galli S, Lissiani A, Gregori A, Bozzola A (2002) Minimally invasive laparoscopic neobladder. J Urol 168(3):1080–1083
14. Gill IS, Kaouk JH, Meraney AM, Desai MM, Vichaker JC, Klein EA, Savage SJ, Sung GT (2002) Laparoscopic radical cystectomy and continent orthotopic ileal neobladder performed completely intracorporeally: the initial experience. J Urol 168(1):13–18
15. Simonato A, Gregori A, Lissiani A, Bozzola A, Galli S, Gaboardi F (2004) Intracorporeal uretero-enteric anastomoses during laparoscopic continent urinary diversion. BJU Int 93(9):1351–1354
16. Abdel-Hakim AM, Bassiouny F, Abdel Azim MS, Rady I, Mohey T, Habib I, Fathi H (2002) Laparoscopic radical cystectomy with orthotopic neobladders. J Endourol 16:377–381
17. Basillote JB, Abdelshehid C, Ahlering TE, Shanberg AM (2004) Laparoscopic assisted radical cystectomy with ileal neobladder: a comparison with the open approach. J Urol 172(2):489–493
18. Hemal AK, Kumar R, Seth A, Gupta NP (2004) Complications of laparoscopic radical cystectomy during the initial experience.Int J Urol 11(7):483–488
19. Hemal AK, Eun D, Tewari A, Menon M (2004) Nuances in the optimum placement of ports in pelvic and upper urinary tract surgery using the da Vinci robot. Urol Clin North Am 31(4):683–692
20. Kaul S, Bhandari A, Hemal AK, Savera A, Shrivastava A, Menon M (2005) Robotic radical prostatectomy with preservation of the prostatic fascia: a feasibility study. Urology: in press
21. Menon M, Hemal AK, Tewari A, Shrivastava A, Shoma AM, El-Tabey NA, Shaaban A, Abol-Enein H, Ghoneim MA (2003) Nerve-sparing robot-assisted radical cystoprostatectomy and urinary diversion. BJU Int 92(3):232–236
22. Menon M, Hemal AK, Tewari A, Shrivastava A, Shoma AM, Abol-Ein H, Ghoneim MA (2004) Robot-assisted radical cystectomy and urinary diversion in female patients: technique with preservation of the uterus and vagina. J Am Coll Surg 198(3):386–393
23. Beecken WD, Wolfram M, Engl T, Bentas W, Probst M, Blaheta R, Oertl A, Jonas D, Binder J (2003) Robotic-assisted laparoscopic radical cystectomy and intra-abdominal formation of an orthotopic ileal neobladder. Eur Urol 44(3):337–339
24. Yohannes P, Puri V, Yi B, Khan AK, Sudan R (2003) Laparoscopy-assisted robotic radical cystoprostatectomy with ileal conduit urinary diversion for muscle-invasive bladder cancer: initial two cases. J Endourol 17(9):729–732
25. Parra RO, Andrus CH, Jones JP (1992) Laparoscopic cystectomy. initial report on a new treatment for the retained bladder. J Urol 148:1140–1144
26. Sanchez de Badajoz E, Gallego Perales JL, Reche Rosado A, Gutierrez de la Cruz JM, Jimenez Garrido A (1995) Laparoscopic cystectomy and ileal conduit: case report. J Endourol 9:59–62
27. Turk I, Deger S, Winkelmann B, Schonberger B, Leoning SA (2001) Laparoscopic radical cystectomy with continent urinary diversion (rectal sigmoid pouch) performed completely intracorporeally: the initial 5 cases. J Urol 165:1863–1866.

Part 4
Prostate

Laparoscopic Radical Prostatectomy: Techniques and Complications

Fernando Pablo Secin, Nicholas Karanikolas, Karim Touijer, and Bertrand Guillonneau

Summary. Laparoscopic radical prostatectomy (LRP) has gained increasing importance in the laparoscopic urologic oncology field and has become an established treatment for localized prostate cancer. The indications for laparoscopic radical prostatectomy are the same as those for the open technique. The advantages of the laparoscopic approach are a magnified view of the anatomic structures and a decreased venous bleeding in the surgical field allowing an accurate dissection of the prostate and neurovascular bundles. The LRP technique is well standardized. Five trocars are used; the patient is placed in the Trendelenburg position. The different steps of the operation are: dissection of the seminal vesicles, via a direct approach, after incising the peritoneum above Douglas' cul-de-sac; creation of a space between the rectum and prostate behind Denonvilliers' fascia; release of the bladder to approach the space of Retzius; opening of the endopelvic fascia and intracorporeal ligature of the dorsal vascular complex; dissection of the prostate from the bladder, by close dissection of the bladder neck; control of the pedicles and dissection of the neurovascular bundles; sectioning of the urethra and removal of the prostate in a bag, urethrovesical anastomosis performed with interrupted intracorporeal sutures, Foley catheter installation; placement of an aspiration drain; and closure. Knowledge of the prostatic anatomy, advanced laparoscopic skills, and expertise in surgical oncology are essential to provide optimal oncologic outcomes while maintaining the highest standards of life quality.

Keywords. Laparoscopy, Prostatectomy, Prostate, Cancer

Department of Urology, Sidney Kimmel Center for Prostate and Urologic Cancers, Memorial Sloan-Kettering Cancer Center, 1275 York Avenue, New York, NY 10021, USA

Introduction

Laparoscopic radical prostatectomy (LRP) has gained increasing importance in the laparoscopic urologic oncology field and has become an established treatment for localized prostate cancer. The initial report of LRP by Schuessler was of nine cases performed through an transperitoneal approach [1]. Shortly thereafter, a single case of a laparoscopic radical prostatectomy through an extraperitoneal approach was reported [2]. However, in the largest initial series originating from France, the transperitoneal approach was used [3–9]. With accrued experience and worldwide use, modifications in the approach and the instrumentation used were introduced [10–16]. This chapter describes antegrade transperitoneal LRP currently performed at Memorial Sloan-Kettering Cancer Center (MSKCC) and reviews its potential complications.

Patient Selection and Preoperative Preparation

The indications for laparoscopic radical prostatectomy are the same as those for the open technique [17]. However, similarly to the open approach, the surgeon often faces different situations that might make the laparoscopic approach more technically challenging. These include obese patients, patients with a large prostate gland, patients whose prostates have a large median lobe, patients with a narrow deep pelvis, those with a history of abdominal/pelvic surgery or pelvic fracture, and those with previous radiotherapy to the pelvis.

No bowel or rectal preparation is needed, but a fleet enema is often recommended for patients. A single dose of a first generation cephalosporin is administrated prior to surgery as antibiotic-prophylaxis [19,20].

Thromboprophylaxis is done by administering 2500 IU of low-molecular-weight heparin subcutaneously 2 h before the operation according to the patient's risk of deep venous thrombosis (DVT). Patients continue to receive this daily dose until they are discharged from the hospital [21,22]. Pneumatic compression stockings are also used during the surgery, and they are discontinued when the patient resumes ambulation [23].

Rationale for Transperitoneal Approach

Both transperitoneal and preperitoneal prostatectomy techniques are now performed for localized prostate cancer at several centers [24,25]. The main advantages of the transperitoneal approach are greater mobilization of the bladder, which allows a tension-free anastomosis, more working space, and a more meticulous dissection of the seminal vesicles (SV). It is our belief that dissecting the

SV first can minimize damage to the pelvic plexus, which is particularly important when a nerve-sparing procedure is planned.

The transperitoneal approach allows faster placement of the trocars. However, the preperitoneal approach eliminates the time associated with the transperitoneal bladder dissection. This method may also reduce even further the minimal but real risk of bladder injury, given that the space of Retzius is developed initially. In addition, once performed, there is little concern regarding visceral injury.

The bowel is in the operative field with the transperitoneal approach and thus, a steeper Trendelenburg position is required to move the bowel out of the pelvic cavity, at least during the initial step, when dissection of the SV is considered.

In the preperitoneal approach the peritoneum isolates the operative field from the abdominal cavity. This method is advantageous, as bleeding, when encountered, does not contact the bowel, thus avoiding reflex ileus. Also, a poor anastomosis does not result in urinary ascites with its associated complications.

The transperitoneal approach does not prevent the patient from receiving adjuvant radiation therapy if required, as all pelvic structures are repositioned to their preoperative anatomical locations. The small bowel does not get interposed between the pubic bone and the bladder postoperatively.

There is an incorrect belief that minimally invasive prostatectomy should mimic what is done in open surgery. Especially when done extraperitoneally, the laparoscopic technique, because of its much improved visualization and working room, may improve on the open prostatectomy technique with better oncological and quality of life results.

The Instruments

The quality of the optic chain (camera and monitor) is important, especially late in the procedure when the anatomical constraints of the deep pelvis limit the quality of the images. The monitors can either be flat LCD (liquid crystal display) panels or conventional CRT (cathode ray tube). The quality of the conventional CRT in terms of color, resolution, brightness, and viewing angle is superior and is our preference.

We perform the laparoscopic radical prostatectomy with mostly reusable material: two axial long prehension forceps, bipolar forceps (one thin, one flat and one triangular), laparoscopic scissors, three 5.5 × 55-mm trocars, one 5.5 × 55-mm trocar with a lateral insufflation valve, one 10-mm trocar, two straight needle holders, one Heggar rectal bougie no. 24, and a Béniqué sound Ch 20. The only disposable material is a 10-mm bag to remove the specimen and a 5-mm suction cannula. In obese patients we use longer trocars (5.5 × 70 mm).

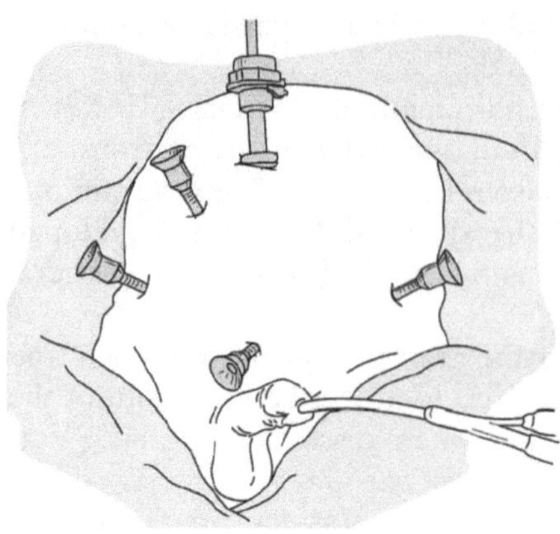

Fig. 1. Disposition of trocars in the abdomen (Modified from Hoznek et al. [17])

Surgical Technique

Transperitoneal pneumoperitoneum is made with the patient in the flat position and set at an intra-abdominal pressure of 12 mmHg. A 10-mm trocar is then inserted into the umbilicus for passage of the 0-degree optic. Next, the patient is positioned in Trendelenburg, so that the small bowel and the sigmoid colon mobilize cephalad to facilitate access to the pelvic region. The height and tilt of the operating table is adjusted to the surgeon's preference. Four 5-mm trocars are inserted: one into the left iliac fossa, one into the midline halfway between the umbilicus and the pubis, one at the level of the umbilicus in the right pararectal line, and the last in the right iliac fossa at Mc Burney's point (Fig. 1).

Standardized steps are classically described.

First Step: Posterior Approach to the Seminal Vesicles

On occasions, the sigmoid colon needs to be detached from the parietal peritoneal fold to allow its complete mobilization out of the Pouch of Douglas and eventually expose the left iliac vessels if a lymph node dissection is to be performed. Once mobilized, the sigmoid colon may be held gently by the assistant with the suction cannula, retracting the rectum superiorly, which facilitates access to the SV dissection (Fig. 2). A 4–5-cm horizontal incision is made approximately 2 cm above the cul de sac on the anterior aspect of the cul-de-sac of Douglas. The dissection should then follow the inferior peritoneal flap. After coagulation of the few sub-peritoneal vessels, the dissection continues into an avascular plane.

Once a sheath of fibrous tissue upholstering the SV complex is identified, the outlines of the seminal vesicles and vasa deferentia are visible. This fascia is transversally incised allowing clear identification of the vasa deferentia. The vas is dissected a few centimeters from the ampulla and coagulated with bipolar

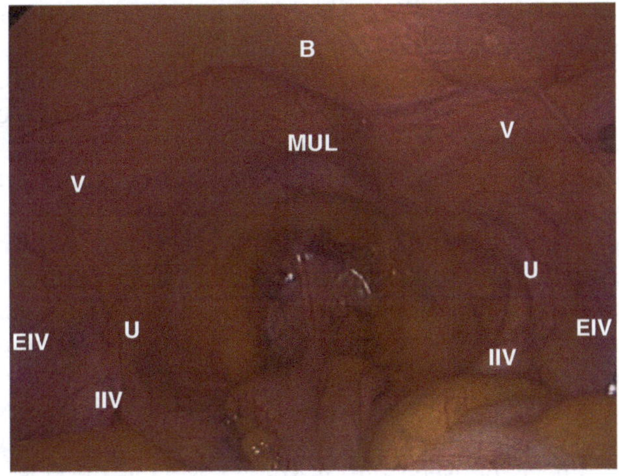

FIG. 2. Laparoscopic anatomy of the pelvic cavity. *U*, ureter; *IIV*, internal iliac vessels; *EIV*, external iliac vessels; *B*, bladder; *MUL*, median umbilical ligament

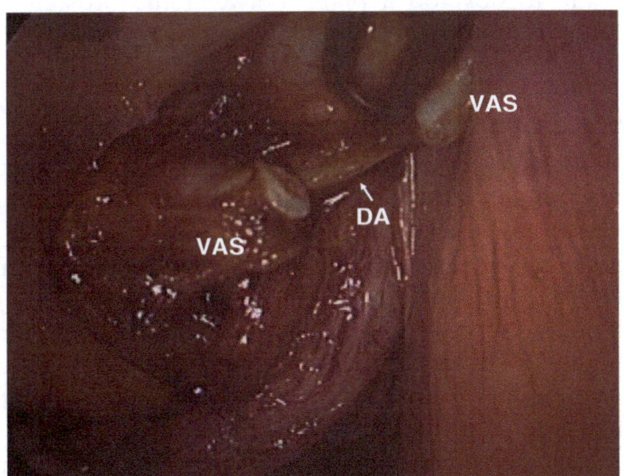

FIG. 3. Deferential artery. *VAS*, vas deferens; *DA*, deferential artery

forceps or clipped and then transected. The deferential artery runs between the vas and the SV, and will not be visible until the vas is sectioned (Fig. 3). This artery is large and can cause serious intra- and postoperative bleeding, so careful coagulation is mandatory. Division of the vas and deferential artery allows access to the seminal vesicle just behind. The assistant's grasping of the prostatic end of the vas facilitates exposure of the posterior aspect of the seminal vesicle. The dissection of the SV should be carried out following a plane along its surface to avoid thermal damage to any surrounding neurological structures.

The posterior aspect of the seminal vesicle is usually nonvascularized and can be easily freed. The anterior aspect of the SV, the one in contact with the bladder, is usually irrigated by one to three arteries.

The dissection of the tip of the seminal vesicle exposes one or two arteries that must be controlled and sectioned to free the seminal vesicle completely. Failure to selectively fulgurate any of these SV arteries may cause significant postoperative hemorrhage.

Once the first SV is dissected (usually the right one), the assistant should pull away the previously dissected and transected vas in order to bring the contralateral vas to the midline and facilitate its dissection. The same surgical strategy for the dissection of the vas and the seminal vesicle is applied to the contralateral side. Then, the assistant retracts both vasa deferentia upwards with a grasper introduced through the suprapubic port to tent Denonvilliers' fascia. The Denonvilliers' fascia is then incised horizontally 1 cm in the midline, where it reflects between the prostatic base and the posterior surface of the seminal vesicles to expose the prerectal fat. This maneuver simplifies the subsequent location of the medial limit of the neurovascular bundles (NVB), as it detaches the prostate from the rectum and prostatic pedicles. No further attempt should be made to develop a plane between the prostate and the rectum posteriorly towards the prostatic apex.

Second Step: Anterior Approach of the Prostate

Before starting the dissection of the retropubic space, the bladder may be filled with approximately 120–180 cc of saline to help identify its contours. It also helps with the dissection, as the weight of the saline pulls the bladder posteriorly. The anterior parietal peritoneum is opened from one medial umbilical ligament to the other in an inverted U-shaped incision. Dissecting laterally and caudally from here, the surgeon locates the pubic arches. The urachus is divided at the end to minimize the risk of bladder injury. It is essential to free the bladder wall from its lateral and anterior attachments in order to create a large working space and to permit a tension-free vesicourethral anastomosis at the end of the operation.

Once the bladder is freed, it should be actively emptied with a syringe as the Trendelenburg position may prevent its complete passive emptying.

The fat of the retropubic space must be swept laterally to expose clearly the, the endopelvic fascia, and the puboprostatic ligaments (Fig. 4). Once the superficial dorsal vein is transected, the fat covering the endopelvic fascia can be easily swept off.

The entire endopelvic fascia is incised laterally on its line of reflection, starting at the level of the base of the prostate and extending anteriorly towards the apex, exposing the levator ani muscle. We identify one or more accessory pudendal arteries (APA) during dissection of either the endopelvic fascia or the puboprostatic ligaments in 30% of cases (in press). This APA should be preserved, since, instead of penetrating into the prostate, it continues parallel to the dorsal vascular complex DVC towards the anterior perineum, and it may

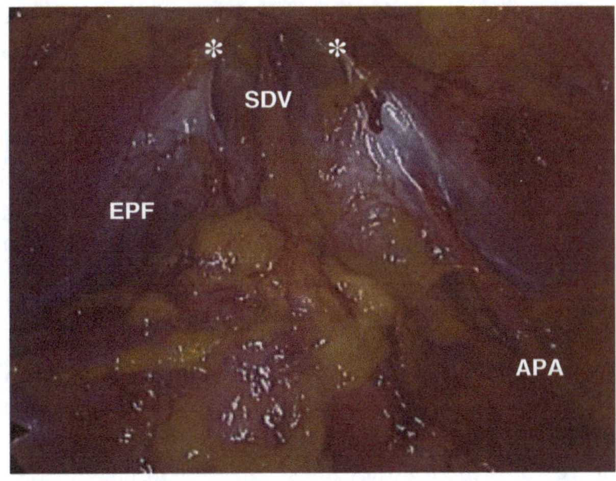

FIG. 4. Endopelvic fascia and puboprostatic ligaments. *SDV*, superficial dorsal vein; *EPF*, endopelvic fascia; *asterisks*, puboprostatic ligaments; *APA*, accessory pudendal artery

have an impact on recovery of potency in patients undergoing nerve sparing surgery.

The DVC is then ligated with a 2-0 polyglactin suture on a #26 SH needle. Depending on the size of the plexus, a second separate suture or a "figure-of-8" stitch may be placed to make the ligation more secure. In the case of bleeding from the DVC, it is of no use to try to control it with any kind of fulguration. Instead, the intra-abdominal pressure can be transiently raised up to 20mmHg while the definitive ligature is placed.

Transection of the complex is not required at this point as it will only cause useless bleeding. This step will be performed later in the operation.

A stitch to prevent back bleeding from the preprostatic veins is placed on the anterior aspect of the prostate. This stitch may be of help during the bladder neck dissection by decreasing the back flow coming from the transected veins on the prostatic side.

Third Step: Bladder Neck Dissection

This step is often felt to be difficult since the anatomical landmarks are not as well defined as in other phases of the surgery. The place where the bladder neck should be dissected is exactly where the fat becomes adherent to the anterior bladder wall. For this area to be recognized, the anterior prevesical fat must be swept off superiorly until it becomes more adherent to the detrusor. This causes a faint outline at the prostatovesical junction, at the exact location where it should be opened. It is generally easy to develop the plane of dissection between bladder and prostate with sharp and blunt dissection. The vesical end of the prostatic urethra is identified by a sudden change in the orientation of the muscular fibers which become longitudinal rather than circular or plexiform. The bladder is emptied again and the catheter balloon deflated.

The bladder neck is incised transversally and the tip of the Foley catheter is pulled upwards with a grasper inserted through the suprapubic port. The scrub nurse pulls this grasper and at the same time places tension by pulling the Foley catheter in order to tent and lift up the prostate and expose the posterior bladder neck wall.

The entire thickness of the posterior bladder neck wall is then incised. This is a step where the dissecting pace should be reduced as this is a highly vascularized area and discrete coagulation alternating the use of the tip of the scissors and the bipolar forceps is needed. The ureteral orifices may be close to the edge of the bladder and their location should always be checked, especially when a median lobe is present, as the bladder mucosa may need to be incised closer to the ureteral orifices in order to achieve a safe oncologic margin.

The correct plane of dissection leads to the recognition of longitudinal bladder muscular fibers tented between the prostate base and the outer layer of the detrusor at the bladder neck. This fibromuscular tissue should be incised in order to gain access to the previously dissected vasa and the seminal vesicles.

The vasa deferentia and the seminal vesicles are then simply brought forward. This maneuver leaves both prostatic pedicles and the edges of the bladder neck lateral to the seminal vesicles.

Fourth Step: Control of the Prostatic Pedicles and Dissection of the NVB

Once the edges of the bladder neck are dissected, lateral to the SV the entire tissue is composed of prostatic pedicle first and the NVB posteriorly. The prostatic pedicle should be taken down with meticulous coagulation with thin bipolars. This procedure is facilitated by anterior traction on the seminal vesicles. Dissection of the NVB can be performed at variable distances from the prostate. The amount of periprostatic tissue removed with the specimen will depend on the characteristics of the tumor, its location and Gleason score, magnetic resonance imaging results, and digital rectal examination.

Keeping this in mind, there are three surgical methods to dissect the NVB (Fig. 5). First, an interfascial technique where the NVB is completely preserved, as the dissection is carried out between the prostatic capsule and the prostatic fascia. Second, an extra technique where the NVB may be partially resected, as the fascia covering the NVB is incised in order to get a wider oncologic margin. Finally, the NVB is resected as the dissection takes place lateral to the NVB.

Fifth Step: Apical Dissection of the Prostate

At this point in the operation, the prostate is anchored by four definite structures: the DVC, the urethra, the distal attachments of the Denonvilliers' fascia to the rectourethralis muscle, and the distal third of both NVB.

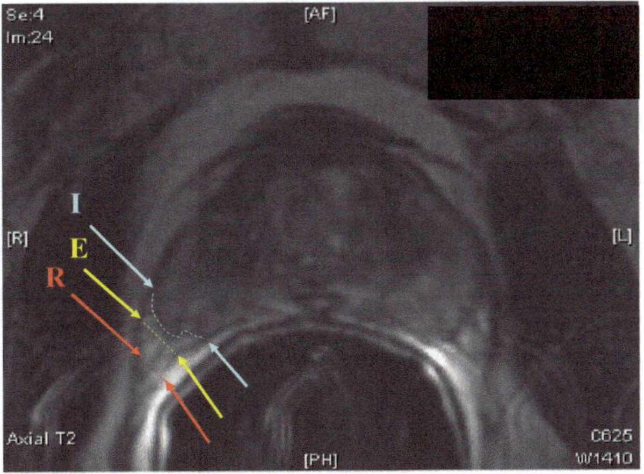

Fig. 5. Planes of neurovascular bundle dissection. *E*, extrafascial; *I*, intrafascial; *R*, resection of the neurovascular bundle

In sequence, we first section the already ligated DVC. The DVC is incised until an avascular plane of dissection between the DVC and the urethra is developed. This plane must be dissected to expose perfectly the anterior and lateral urethral walls. A Béniqué sound is introduced to help identify the urethra by improving the tactile perception of its limits. Next, we complete the dissection of the distal third of the neurovascular bundles. During this step, excessive traction on the prostate should be avoided so as not to stretch the urethra and the sphincteric complex.

Then, once the NVBs have been dissected from the apex, the distal attachments of Denonvilliers' fascia are incised on both sides. It is individualized at the apex and dissected from the posterior aspect of the urethra. Finally, after the prostate has been freed from all these structures, it will be left hanging from the urethra, and is incised with cold scissors. We have observed that leaving the urethra for the end decreases the chance of positive surgical margins at the apex.

Once the specimen is free, a 5-mm scope is inserted through a lateral port and the gland is placed into the 10-mm laparoscopic bag. The umbilical incision is extended at the midline according to the size of the gland and the specimen is extracted. The gland is macroscopically examined for the presence of induration, nodularity, or an area suspicious for positive margin that could require confirmation by frozen section examination. When in doubt of a positive surgical margin, we recommend submitting the entire gland for pathologic evaluation, tagging the suspicious areas with a 6-0 stitch. Evaluation of a possible positive margin should not be done from a second sample of tissue taken from the prostatic bed. In the event of a pathologic confirmation of a positive surgical margin, additional tissue is to be resected.

The umbilical fascia is carefully closed with two running 0 sutures starting at each edge and tightened (not tied) around a 10-mm trocar. Then the abdomen is reinsufflated. The pelvis is inspected and any clots are aspirated and the pelvis is irrigated with saline at 37°C temperature. Hemostasis is confirmed. Always include inspection of the SV lodge, the prostatic pedicles and the NVBs, as these are the most frequent locations of bleeding.

Sixth Step: Urethrovesical Anastomosis

We never evert the bladder mucosa and we do not reconstruct a large bladder neck opening before the anastomosis is done. An anterior tennis racquet is usually performed at the end if needed. In more than 400 cases followed prospectively, we found only one case of bladder neck contracture (BNC) secondary to a pelvic hematoma.

Ten interrupted stitches of 3-0 polyglactin suture with a #18-mm half-circle needle are used for the anastomosis. All knots are tied intracorporeally. The Béniqué sound not only helps to guide the needle into the urethral lumen but also to take the full thickness of the urethral wall with the stitch.

The three first sutures are placed posteriorly at 5, 6, and 7 o'clock, going inside-out on the urethra and outside-in on the bladder neck. The 5 o'clock stitch goes inside-out on the urethra (right hand, forehand) and outside-in on the bladder (right hand, forehand); the 6 and 7 o'clock stitches go inside-out on the urethra (right hand, forehand) and outside-in on the bladder (left hand, forehand). These stitches are therefore tied intraluminally, and in our experience this has not been associated with calcifications, lithiasis, or BNC.

Four other sutures are symmetrically placed at 4 and 8, then 2 and 10 o'clock, and tied outside the lumen. The sutures at 4 and 2 o'clock go outside-in on the bladder (right hand, forehand) and inside-out on the urethra (left hand, backhand). The sutures at 8 and 10 o'clock go outside-in on the bladder (left hand, forehand) and inside-out on the urethra (right hand, backhand).

Three final anterior stitches are placed at 11, 12, and 1 o'clock, symmetrically to the posterior stitches. The 11 and 12 o'clock stitches go outside-in on the urethra (right hand, forehand) and inside-out on the bladder (right hand, forehand) while the 1 o'clock stitch goes outside-in on the urethra (right hand, forehand) and inside-out on the bladder (left hand, forehand). Once the stitches are tied, the Foley catheter is inserted. The bladder is filled with 180 cc of saline to check for water tightness of the anastomosis and confirm the correct position of the catheter. Finally, the balloon is inflated with 10 ml of sterile water.

The urethrovesical anastomosis can also be accomplished with a running suture, which may be less demanding but which may theoretically reduce the lumen of the anastomosis [26]. The reader is referred to this citation for technical details.

Seventh Step: Completing the Operation and Drainage

The abdominal pressure is lowered to 5 mmHg, to check for venous bleeding. One or two suction drains are placed, one anteriorly in the retropubic space, and one posteriorly, between the rectum and the bladder. The 5-mm trocars are removed under visual control and the parietal orifices are checked to exclude any vascular injury, particularly of the epigastric vessels. At the end, the two running sutures are tied together to close the fascial layer of the umbilical incision. Four-0 running subcuticular Poliglecaprone is used in all port incisions.

Postoperative Care

For pain management, patients are initially given morphine sulfate in the recovery room 2–5 mg i.v. q 2 h as needed + Ketorolac 15 mg i.v. q 6 h for a maximum of six doses. When patients can tolerate fluids orally, Oxycodone 5 mg with acetaminophen 325 mg replaces the previous medications.

Patients are requested to ambulate with assistance on the night of the surgery and then without it the following day until discharge.

Patients are given clear fluids 6 h after surgery and a light breakfast the following morning. Diet is progressed to regular if adequately tolerated.

The Foley catheter is removed on postoperative day 7. Cystograms are not routinely performed.

Kegel exercises are started 3 days after catheter removal [27–29].

Patients usually start passing gases on postoperative day 2 and have their first bowel movement on postoperative day 3. It is recommended that they avoid abundant meals until after they start moving bowels.

Drinking fluids is encouraged while patients have the Foley catheter in place; however, fluid may be decreased to what they normally drink after the Foley catheter is removed.

Full exercise, including sexual activity, may be resumed after 3 weeks of surgery [30–32].

Complications and Management [33]

Intraoperative Complications

Bleeding from the DVC

Although laparoscopy allows a clear vision of the apex, and the pneumoperitoneum provides a tamponade effect, bleeding from the DVC can be significant and may affect the remainder of the operation due to impaired visibility. A meticulous apical dissection defining the principal anatomical elements around the DVC is essential to preventing unnecessary hemorrhage.

When the ligating suture is loose, placed too proximal, or cut during the transection of the DVC, bleeding can be controlled either by increasing the pneumoperitoneum pressure up to 20 mmHg. or by clamping the DVC with a grasper. This allows a tamponade effect while the surgeon is calmly preparing a second ligating suture. Once tied, the DVC stitch can be anchored to the periosteum of the pubic symphysis.

Bladder Injury

The bladder is more likely to be inadvertently damaged at three different times during transperitoneal laparoscopic radical prostatectomy. First, during the posterior dissection of the seminal vesicles: dissection in fatty tissue should alert the surgeon of a plane either too close to the bladder or to the rectum. Second, during the development of the retropubic space: any excessive bleeding should alert the surgeon of a dissection too close to the bladder. Third, during the dissection of the posterior bladder neck: the area at risk is the trigone and retrotrigonal bladder wall. On identification, the surgeon should verify the integrity of the ureters and ureteral orifices and repair the bladder with resorbable suture.

Rectal Injury

Rectal injuries most frequently occur during prostate dissection at the apex. They may result from a direct cut into the rectal wall, or from a microperforation secondary to thermal injury due to excessive cauterization on the rectal wall surface [34]. The risk of rectal injury increases when there is a substantial amount of periprostatic inflammatory reaction, prior prostate surgery or radiation, a large volume gland with a narrow pelvis, non-nerve sparing LRP, and surgeon's inexperience. Intraoperative rectal examination with the finger, rectal bougie or balloon might be of help to prevent or identify rectal injuries while incising Denonvilliers' fascia and dissecting the posterior surface of the prostate.

If an incision on the rectal wall is recognized, it is generally accepted that the defect can be sutured primarily with a two layers of interrupted 2-0 silk after débridement of any devitalized tissue if no gross fecal soiling is observed. Interposition of an omental flap or pararectal fat flap is not routinely necessary. However, in face of a large, devitalized rectal laceration or of gross soiling, a temporary diverting colostomy is advisable.

Microperforations of the rectal wall often go unrecognized until after the Foley catheter is removed and is manifested by a rectourethral fistula. The first therapeutic option is to reinsert the Foley catheter until the fistula heals spontaneously. If this conservative method fails, elective surgical approach of the recto-urethral fistula should be considered. Needless to say, prevention is the mainstay of therapy.

Ureter Injury

This may occur either during the dissection of the seminal vesicles by mistakenly sectioning the ureter instead of the vas deferens, or by an inadvertent thermal injury. When the injury is not identified intraoperatively, a persistent urine leakage or uroperitoneum with a watertight anastomosis suggests the diagnosis. Ureteral reimplantation is the treatment of choice. Another reported ureteral complication is a postoperative anuria caused by incorporation of the ureteral orifices in the urethrovesical anastomotic sutures. If identified while the patient is in hospital, the anastomosis should be redone laparoscopically.

Epigastric Artery Injury

Because of anatomy, the epigastrics are more frequently injured while placing the right paramedial port. Bleeding around the trocar, either internally or externally, suggests a vessel injury. Placement of the port lateral to the rectus abdominis muscle is safer. Venous injury can be managed successfully by tamponade, whereas arterial injury requires surgical hemostasis using the Reverdin or the Carter-Thomason needle. As a fundamental rule of laparoscopic surgery, all the trocars should be removed under direct vision with decreased abdominal pressure.

Postoperative Complications

Urine Leakage

An increased and prolonged urine output from the pelvic drain suggests the diagnosis. In the majority of cases, the left posterior aspect of the anastomosis is compromised and is managed conservatively by prolonging both bladder and pelvic drainage. If the leak persists despite a conservative treatment, a ureteral injury or an eversion of the ureteral orifice outside of the anastomosis needs to be ruled out.

On occasions, the urinary leak may be diagnosed after the catheter is removed. In patients with transperitoneal radical prostatectomy, the sudden onset of sharp abdominal pain during or immediately after urination is a urinary leak until proven otherwise. The treatment consists of reinsertion of the catheter and reassessment of the anastomosis by a retrograde cystogram at a later date to ascertain a complete healing of the anastomosis. We advocate obtaining a urinalysis before any manipulation to identify and treat any urinary tract infection and limit the risk of uroperitonitis.

Small Bowel Injury

The small bowel can be injured either early in the operation during trocar placement or by thermal injury during prostate dissection. A missed bowel injury will manifest by ileus, increased abdominal pain, and decreased white blood cell counts with or without signs of systemic infection. Prompt computed tomography scan imaging with oral contrast may lead to the diagnosis. Therapy requires a re-exploration, which can be done laparoscopically.

Nerve Compression and Compartment Syndrome

Ulnar and brachial neuropraxia have been reported following LRP and have resulted in a transient paresis. This type of complication is related to patient positioning. One way to prevent it is by avoiding narrow operating room tables so that the operating surgeon does not inadvertently lean on the patient's arm.

We prefer the low lithotomy position because it allows easy access to the rectum if needed. However, lithotomy position for long periods of time may lead to compartment syndrome: a potential complication that should always be ruled out postoperatively. Over-tightness of the calves by the sequential compressive devices and stirrups might contribute to this syndrome. Distal pulses should always be assessed pre and postoperatively as well as distal capillary refill at the nail beds, as it usually precedes cessation of arterial flow. Myoglobinuria, electrolyte disturbances, disorders of acid–base balance, and serum creatine kinase values of over 2000 U/l after surgery may be considered a warning sign in ventilated and sedated patients, in whom early clinical symptoms of compartment syndrome, such as pain and paresthesias, cannot be ascertained [35]. The treatment is emergent fasciotomy of the muscular groups involved.

Obturator nerve neuropraxia is usually associated with LND. It is manifested by different degrees of postoperative throbbing, unrelenting leg pain, and weakness. Abducting capacity of the leg is markedly diminished and more frequently takes place on the left side due to the greater difficulty of the LND on this side [36,37].

In the presence of postoperative leg pain, think first of acute compartment syndrome, particularly if symptoms are bilateral, outside the abductor muscle territory, and in a patient in whom LND had not been performed.

Conclusions

Laparoscopic radical prostatectomy is a relatively new approach to the surgical treatment of localized prostate cancer. Since its inception, the technique, however challenging, is undergoing continuous refinements which make it today a feasible, reproducible, and teachable operation practiced by urologists worldwide. The advantages of the laparoscopic approach are a magnified view of the anatomic structures, and decreased venous bleeding in the surgical field to allow an accurate dissection of the prostate and neurovascular bundles. Theses advantages should translate to better outcomes, in term of cancer control and functional results.

References

1. Schuessler WW, Schulam PG, Clayman RV, Kavoussi LR (1997) Laparoscopic radical prostatectomy: initial short-term experience. Urology 50:854–857

2. Raboy A, Ferzli G, Albert P (1997) Initial experience with extraperitoneal endoscopic radical retropubic prostatectomy. Urology 50:849–853
3. Guillonneau B, Cathelineau X, Barret E, Rozet F, Vallancien G (1998) [Laparoscopic radical prostatectomy. Preliminary evaluation after 28 interventions]. Presse Med 27:1570–1574
4. Guillonneau B, Cathelineau X, Barret E, Rozet F, Vallancien G (1999) Laparoscopic radical prostatectomy: technical and early oncological assessment of 40 operations. Eur Urol 36:14–20
5. Guillonneau B, Cathelineau X, Doublet JD, Baumert H, Vallancien G (2002) Laparoscopic radical prostatectomy: assessment after 550 procedures. Crit Rev Oncol Hematol 43:123–133
6. Guillonneau B, Cathelineau X, Doublet JD, Vallancien G (2001) Laparoscopic radical prostatectomy: the lessons learned. J Endourol 15:441–445; discussion 447–448
7. Guillonneau B, el-Fettouh H, Baumert H, Cathelineau X, Doublet JD, Fromont G, Vallancien G (2003) Laparoscopic radical prostatectomy: oncological evaluation after 1,000 cases at Montsouris Institute. J Urol 169:1261–1266
8. Guillonneau B, Rozet F, Barret E, Cathelineau X, Vallancien G (2001) Laparoscopic radical prostatectomy: assessment after 240 procedures. Urol Clin North Am 28:189–202
9. Vallancien G, Guillonneau B, Cathelineau X, Baumert H, Doublet JD (2002) [Localized prostatic cancer: treatment with laparoscopic radical prostatectomy: study with 841 cases]. Bull Acad Natl Med 186:117–123; discussion 123–114
10. Bollens R, Vanden Bossche M, Roumeguere T, Damoun A, Ekane S, Hoffmann P, Zlotta AR, Schulman CC (2001) Extraperitoneal laparoscopic radical prostatectomy. Results after 50 cases. Eur Urol 40:65–69
11. Dubernard P, Benchetrit S, Chaffange P, Hamza T, Van Box Som P (2003) [Retrograde extraperitoneal laparoscopic prostatectomy (R.E.I.P). Simplified technique (based on a series of 143 cases)]. Prog Urol 13:163–174
12. Hoznek A, Antiphon P, Borkowski T, Gettman MT, Katz R, Salomon L, Zaki S, de la Taille A, Abbou CC (2003) Assessment of surgical technique and perioperative morbidity associated with extraperitoneal versus transperitoneal laparoscopic radical prostatectomy. Urology 61:617–622
13. Rassweiler J, Marrero R, Hammady A, Erdogru T, Teber D, Frede T (2004) Transperitoneal laparoscopic radical prostatectomy: ascending technique. J Endourol 18:593–599; discussion 599–600
14. Rassweiler J, Sentker L, Seemann O, Hatzinger M, Rumpelt HJ (2001) Laparoscopic radical prostatectomy with the Heilbronn technique: an analysis of the first 180 cases. J Urol 166:2101–2108
15. Stolzenburg JU, Do M, Pfeiffer H, Konig F, Aedtner B, Dorschner W (2002) The endoscopic extraperitoneal radical prostatectomy (EERPE): technique and initial experience. World J Urol 20:48–55
16. Stolzenburg JU, Do M, Rabenalt R, Pfeiffer H, Horn L, Truss MC, Jonas U, Dorschner W (2003) Endoscopic extraperitoneal radical prostatectomy: initial experience after 70 procedures. J Urol 169:2066–2071
17. Touijer AK, Guillonneau B (2004) Laparoscopic radical prostatectomy. Urol Oncol Semin Orig Invest 22:133–138
18. Dellinger EP, Gross PA, Barrett TL, Krause PJ, Martone WJ, McGowan JE Jr, Sweet RL, Wenzel RP (1994) Quality standard for antimicrobial prophylaxis in surgical pro-

cedures. The Infectious Diseases Society of America. Infect Control Hosp Epidemiol 15:182–188
19. Waddell TK, Rotstein OD (1994) Antimicrobial prophylaxis in surgery. Committee on Antimicrobial Agents, Canadian Infectious Disease Society. Cmaj 151:925–931
20. Colwell CW Jr (2003) Dosing and timing of low-molecular-weight heparin thromboprophylaxis in total hip arthroplasty. Orthopedics 26:1155–1161; quiz 1162–1153
21. Howard PA (1997) Dalteparin: a low-molecular-weight heparin. Ann Pharmacother 31:192–203
22. Beebe DS, McNevin MP, Crain JM, Letourneau JG, Belani KG, Abrams JA, Goodale RL (1993) Evidence of venous stasis after abdominal insufflation for laparoscopic cholecystectomy. Surg Gynecol Obstet 176:443–447
23. Cathelineau X, Cahill D, Widmer H, Rozet F, Baumert H, Vallancien G, Joseph JV, Patel HR (2004) Transperitoneal or extraperitoneal approach for laparoscopic radical prostatectomy: a false debate over a real challenge. J Urol 171:714–716
24. Joseph JV, Patel HR (2004) Transperitoneal or extraperitoneal approach for laparoscopic radical prostatectomy: a false debate over a real challenge. J Urol 172:1545
25. Van Velthoven RF, Ahlering TE, Peltier A, Skarecky DW, Clayman RV (2003) Technique for laparoscopic running urethrovesical anastomosis: the single knot method. Urology 61:699–702
26. Hunter KF, Moore KN, Cody DJ, Glazener CM (2004) Conservative management for postprostatectomy urinary incontinence. Cochrane Database Syst Rev: CD001843
27. Moul JW (1998) Pelvic muscle rehabilitation in males following prostatectomy. Urol Nurs 18:296–301
28. Van Kampen M, De Weerdt W, Van Poppel H, De Ridder D, Feys H, Baert L (2000) Effect of pelvic-floor re-education on duration and degree of incontinence after radical prostatectomy: a randomised controlled trial. Lancet 355:98–102
29. Raina R, Lakin MM, Agarwal A, Sharma R, Goyal KK, Montague DK, Klein E, Zippe CD (2003) Long-term effect of sildenafil citrate on erectile dysfunction after radical prostatectomy: 3-year follow-up. Urology 62:110–115
30. Zippe CD, Kedia AW, Kedia K, Nelson DR, Agarwal A (1998) Treatment of erectile dysfunction after radical prostatectomy with sildenafil citrate (Viagra). Urology 52:963–966
31. Zippe CD, Raina R, Thukral M, Lakin MM, Klein EA, Agarwal A (2001) Management of erectile dysfunction following radical prostatectomy. Curr Urol Rep 2:495–503
32. Guillonneau B, Rozet F, Cathelineau X, Lay F, Barret E, Doublet JD, Baumert H, Vallancien G (2002) Perioperative complications of laparoscopic radical prostatectomy: the Montsouris 3-year experience. J Urol 167:51–56
33. Guillonneau B, Gupta R, El Fettouh H, Cathelineau X, Baumert H, Vallancien G (2003) Laparoscopic management of rectal injury during laparoscopic radical prostatectomy. J Urol 169:1694–1696
34. Lampert R, Weih EH, Breucking E, Kirchhoff S, Lazica B, Lang K (1995) Postoperative bilateral compartment syndrome resulting from prolonged urological surgery in lithotomy position. Serum creatine kinase activity (CK) as a warning signal in sedated, artificially respirated patients. Anaesthesist 44:43–47
35. Arai Y, Egawa S, Terachi T, Suzuki K, Gotoh M, Kawakita M, Tanaka M, Terada N, Baba S, Okumura K, Hayami S, Ono Y, Matsuda T, Naito S (2003) Morbidity of

laparoscopic radical prostatectomy: summary of early multi-institutional experience in Japan. Int J Urol 10:430–434

36. Spaliviero M, Steinberg AP, Kaouk JH, Desai MM, Hammert WC, Gill IS (2004) Laparoscopic injury and repair of obturator nerve during radical prostatectomy. Urology 64:1030

Laparoscopic Radical Prostatectomy: Oncological and Functional Results

Toshiro Terachi[1], Yukio Usui[1], Masanori Shima[1], and Kazuhiro Okumura[2]

Summary. Between December 1999 and December 2004, 160 patients with organ-confined prostate cancer underwent laparoscopic radical prostatectomy (LRP) by two surgeons with many different assistants. The patients were divided into two groups in order of the date of surgery. Groups I and II consisted of 66 and 94 patients who were operated on between December 1999 and March 2002 and between April 2002 and December 2004, respectively. Group I was subdivided into Group I-a and Group I-b: Group I-a consisted of 36 patients who underwent LRP at Tenri Hospital and Group I-b consisted of 30 patients who underwent LRP at the other institutions in the same period. The patients in Group I-b were evaluated only for operative morbidity and excluded from analysis of oncological outcome because of insufficient pathological data. Mean operative time and mean blood loss including leaked urine in Group II were 291 ± 57.2 min (range 145–425 min) and 401.0 ± 323.7 g (range 14–1859 g). There was no blood transfusion in Group II and no operative conversion to an open retropubic radical prostatectomy (RRP). Mean postoperative urethral catheter indwelling period and mean postoperative hospital stay were 4 ± 4.8 days (range 3–28) and 8 ± 4.5 days (range 4–25) in Group II, respectively. Positive surgical margin was detected in 18/130 cases (13.8%) for all pathological stages in this series, but 7/105 cases (6.6%) with pT2 and pT0 disease. Positive surgical margin was detected at the apical margin most frequently. To achieve earlier recovery of urinary continence, a ligation of the dorsal vein complex (DVC bunching) was decided against and substituted by closure of DVC stump with a vertical running suture for hemostasis. In the latter group in Group II, 55% and 87% of the patients were almost dry at 1 and 3 months postoperatively, respectively. Eight of 31 patients (25.8%) who had preserved unilateral neurovascular bundle (NVB) regained potency to be able to carry out sexual intercourse between 6

[1] Department of Urology, Tokai University School of Medicine, Bohseidai, Isehara, Kanagawa 259-1193, Japan
[2] Department of Urology, Tenri Hospital, Tenri, Nara 632-0015, Japan

and 15 months postoperatively. Less morbidity, encouraging early oncological results and improved early recovery of urinary continence, are favorable factors for LRP; however, long-term follow-up and consecutive effort to improve the apical section procedure are required for establishment of LRP as a reliable treatment tool for organ-confined prostate cancer.

Keywords. Laparoscopic radical prostatectomy, Operative modification, Oncological results, Functional results

Introduction

The first laparoscopic radical prostatectomy (LRP) was performed in 1991 by Schuessler et al. [1] before being renewed by Guillonneau et al. in 1998 [2]. Now many series of LRP have been reported from worldwide institutions and more than 3000 procedures have accumulated in the literature [3]. While undertaking a large number of cumulative procedures in a single institution is difficult in Japan because of the low incidence of prostate cancer, a learning curve effect became clear even with a limited experience [4]. After overcoming the complications in early series of LRP, simultaneous control of both oncological and functional results is the object of establishing the LRP procedure as a tool for treatment option of localized prostate cancer. In this chapter we present our perioperative results, pathological evaluation of the removed specimen, functional results, and the modifications of the procedure used to obtain better results in our LRP series of 160 patients.

Materials and Methods

Between December 1999 and December 2004, a total of 160 patients underwent LRP by two surgeons with many different assistants. The indication for radical prostatectomy was a diagnosis of clinically localized prostate cancer (except for two patients with clinical stage T3a disease after several months of neoadjuvant hormone therapy). The patients were divided into two groups in order of the date of surgery. Groups I and II consisted of 66 and 94 patients who were operated on between December 1999 and March 2002 and between April 2002 and December 2004, respectively. Group I was subdivided into Groups I-a and I-b: Group I-a consisted of 36 patients who underwent LRP at Tenri Hospital and Group I-b consisted of 30 patients who underwent LRP at the other institutions in the same period. The patients in Group I-b were evaluated only for operative morbidity and excluded from analysis of oncological outcome because of insufficient pathological data. The age, preoperative prostate-specific antigen (PSA) level, Gleason score of biopsy cores, and preoperative clinical stage of Group I-a and Group II are shown in Fig. 1a–d.

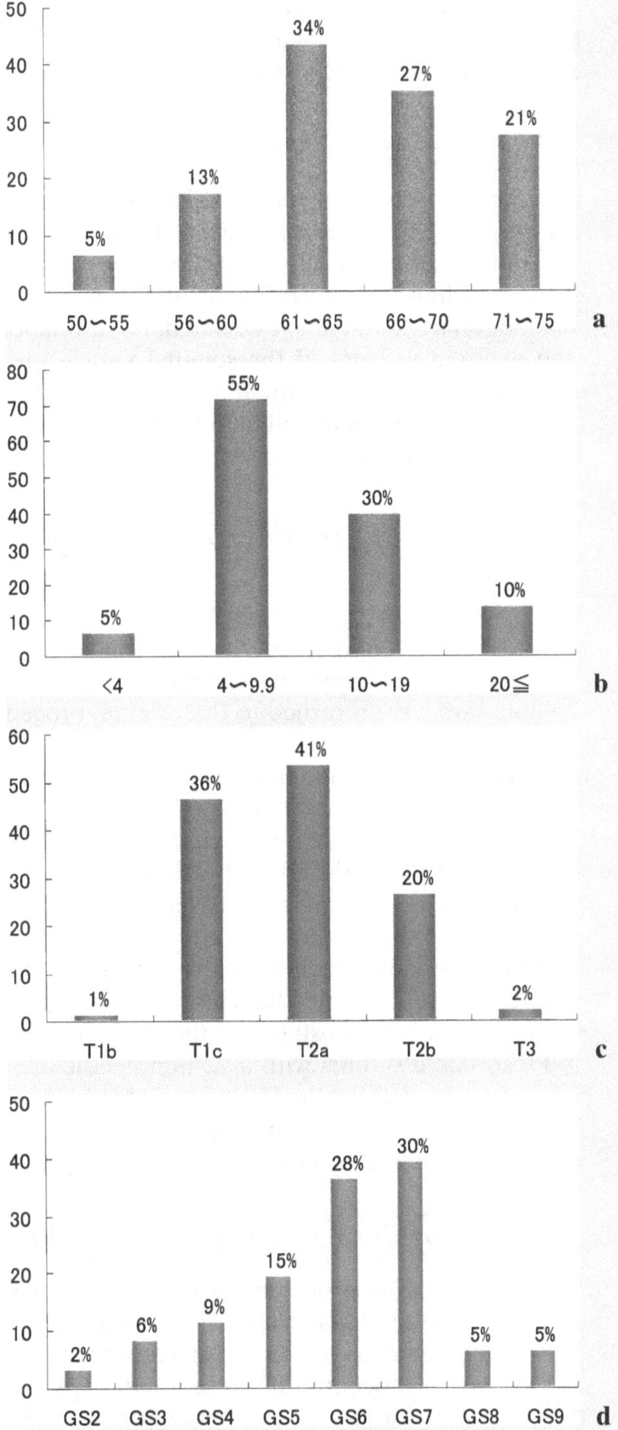

FIG. 1a–d. Patient characteristics of Groups I-a and II. **a** Ages of the patients in Groups I-a and II. **b** Prostate-specific antigen (*PSA*) levels of the patients in Groups I-a and II. **c** Clinical stages of the patients in Groups I-a and II. **d** Gleason scores of the patients in Groups I-a and II

We followed the operative technique of Montsouris [5] initially, but several modifications were added to it after some experience. Our initial procedure is detailed in a previous article [4]. Modifications are as follows.

Dissection of the Seminal Vesicle

The dissection of the seminal vesicle is performed transperitoneally as shown in the original Montsouris technique. In the nerve-sparing procedure the seminal vesicular arteries are clipped proximally before severing without using electrocautery. When the central zone of the prostate protrudes enormously in the bladder on a sagittal image of magnetic resonance imaging (MRI), it is dissected and exposed in front of the seminal vesicle in this step. The adenoma can be easily palpated as an elastic-hard mass by a tip of forceps in front of the seminal vesicle. This procedure will help the precise division of the bladder neck and the protruding prostate.

Division of the Bladder Neck and the Prostate

Converting to retroperitoneal approach to the Retzius cavity using balloon dissection following transperitoneal dissection of the seminal vesicle had been chosen to avoid bladder and vesical vessels injuries in our early experience of the original Montsouris technique. But now with more knowledge of the anatomy we have returned to the original procedure in order to avoid unnecessary time and cost.

Incision of the endopelvic fascia is minimized in the distal portion so as not to damage the pudendal vessels (since November 2004). The levator ani muscle attached to the prostate is dissected with the fascial structure of connective tissue laterally, but the periurethral portion of the muscle is left untouched. The puboprostatic ligaments are not incised and the dorsal vein complex (DVC) is not ligated above the urethra. The endopelvic fascia over the prostate and the anterior fibromuscular stroma (AFS) are ligated together using a 2-0 resorbable suture with a 32-mm needle. This suture is helpful to expose the faint outline of the junction of the prostate and the bladder neck. Three hemostatic sutures with 3-0 resorbable sutures with a 22-mm needle are placed on the bladder neck to prevent unnecessary blood loss during bladder neck division (Fig. 2). The bladder neck is preserved as much as possible for the patients without positive biopsy cores in the prostatic base.

Division of the Lateral Pedicle of the Prostate

The nerve-sparing procedure is performed for those patients with T1c or T2a disease, but only unilaterally for the negative biopsy cores side in most cases. Ten-millimeter clips are used for control of bleeding around the NVB in the nerve-sparing procedure because 5-mm clips drop easily during the dissection. Most recently a laparoscopic bulldog forceps with a following hemostatic running suture has been used instead of clips.

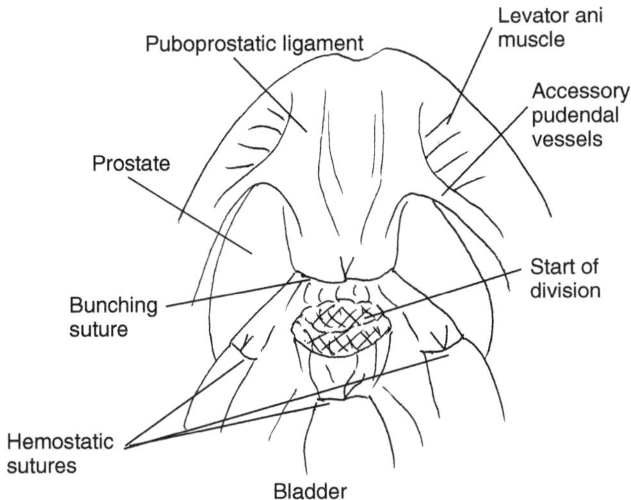

FIG. 2. Division of the prostate and the bladder neck. Three hemostatic sutures are placed on the bladder neck

Apical Section

The first modification in this step, in April 2003, was forgoing a deep DVC ligation above the urethra (DVC bunching) to avoid damage on the urethral sphincter and achieve earlier recovery of urinary continence. Closure of the distal DVC stump using a vertical running suture is performed for hemostasis instead of DVC bunching. The second modification, first done in November 2004, is preservation of the accessory pudendal vessels and the periurethral structures to obtain earliest recovery of urinary continence. The DVC is ligated using only a 2-0 resolvable suture with a 32-mm 3/8 weak curved needle to expose the lateral surface of prostatic apex, proximally to the puboprostatic ligaments and the entrance of the pudendal vessels into the DVC. Division of the DVC is started proximally at the entrance of the pudendal vessels after placing an anchor suture with a 3-0 resorbable suture on the puboprostatic ligament. Bleeding from the DVC is controlled by closure of the distal DVC stump using a vertical running suture of the previous anchor suture (Fig. 3). Dissection of the apex is performed anteriorly and laterally after incising the lateral pelvic fascia on the apex while preserving the periurethral structures. The urethra is incised by electrocautery while keeping the distance between the urethra and the rectum.

Urethrovesical Anastomosis

Urethrovesical anastomosis was performed in the initial 30 patients by eight interrupted sutures in the same manner as in the Montsouris technique. After that, a 3-0 Vicryl running suture with a 26-mm 5/8 strong curved needle was used.

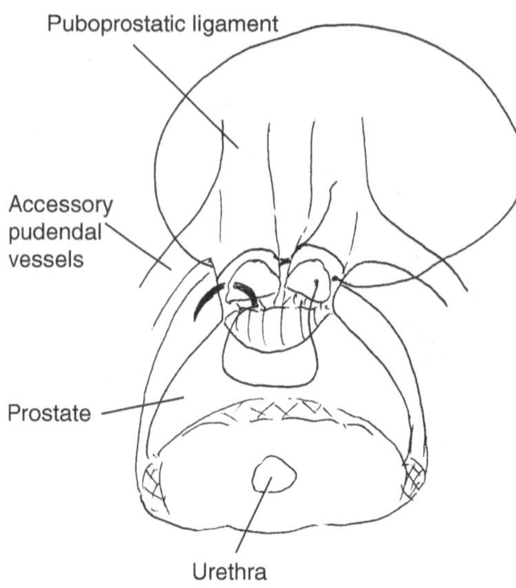

Fig. 3. Division of the dorsal vein complex (DVC). The puboprostatic ligaments and the pudendal vessels are preserved. The distal stump of the DVC is approximated by a vertical running suture for hemostasis

This was changed to the combined procedure with a running suture from 3 to 9 o'clock and three or four interrupted sutures of 10, 12, (1), and 2 o'clock after the first change of apical section procedure. The interrupted sutures on the upper portion of the urethra are fixed to the DVC stump to lift up the bladder neck slightly. Recently the anastomosis returned to seven to nine interrupted sutures with fixation of upper-half sutures to the DVC stump as in the previous procedure. Every suture runs inside out on the urethra to take the required minimum length of the urethral stump.

Results

Perioperative Results

There was no surgical conversion to an open retropubic radical prostatectomy (RRP) in this series. Mean operative time and mean blood loss including leaked urine in Group II were 291 ± 57.2 min (range 145–425 min) and 401.0 ± 323.7 g (range 14–1859 g) against 356 ± 157 min and 364 ± 50 g of the first 30 procedures in Group I [4]. There was no blood transfusion in Group II, but two patients in Group I required homologous blood transfusion adding to autologous blood transfusion. There were no postoperative deaths and thromboembolic complications in this series.

There were four cases (2.5%) of bladder injury, two (1.3%) of rectal injury, two (1.3%) of urethral injury, and one (0.6%) of ureteral injury in addition to seven (4.4%) of hypogastric arterial injury as intraoperative complications in the

TABLE 1. Operative complications

	Group I	Group II
Bladder injury	3	1
Rectal injury	2	0
Urethral injury	1	1
Ureteral injury	1	0

TABLE 2. Postoperative complications

	Group I	Group II
Anastomotic failure	5	2
Urethral stricture	2	1
Postoperative bleeding	2	0
Hydronephrosis	1	1
Rectal perforation	1	0
Rectourethral fistula	1	0
Pubic bone myelitis	1	0
Acute renal failure	0	1
Paralytic ileus	1	0

series (Table 1). All of the injuries were corrected during LRP. Postoperative complications included seven cases (4.4%) of urethrovesical anastomotic failure (urine leakage more than 3 weeks), three (1.9%) of urethral stricture requiring intervention, two (1.3%) of postoperative bleeding, two (1.3%) of hydronephrosis, and one each (0.6%) of rectal perforation, rectourethral fistula, pubic bone myelitis, acute renal failure, and paralytic ileus in the series (Table 2). Reintervention was required in each case of postoperative bleeding from the NVB, rectal perforation and rectourethral fistula.

Mean postoperative urethral catheter indwelling period was 4 ± 4.8 days (range 3–28 days) in Group II against 11.6 ± 9.2 days in the first 30 cases in Group I. Mean postoperative hospital stay was 8 ± 4.5 days (range 4–25 days) in Group II against 19.5 ± 9.1 days in the first 30 cases in Group I.

Oncological Results

Limited lymphadenectomy of the obturator fossa was performed only for the patients with more than 10 ng/ml of PSA level and/or Gleason score of greater than 7. No lymph node metastasis was detected in this series. Pathological examination revealed pT0 disease in 8 patients (5.2%), pT2a disease in 39 (30.0%), pT2b disease in 58 (44.6%), pT3a disease in 19 (14.6%), and pT3b disease in 6 (4.6%). Positive surgical margin (PSM) was detected in 18/130 cases (13.8%) for all pathological stages in this series, but 7/105 cases (6.6%) in pT2 and pT0 disease. Locations of positive surgical margin were dw(+) in 38%, pw(+) in 6%, cap(+) in 28%, dw(+) and cap(+) in 17%, and pw(+) and cap(+) in 11%.

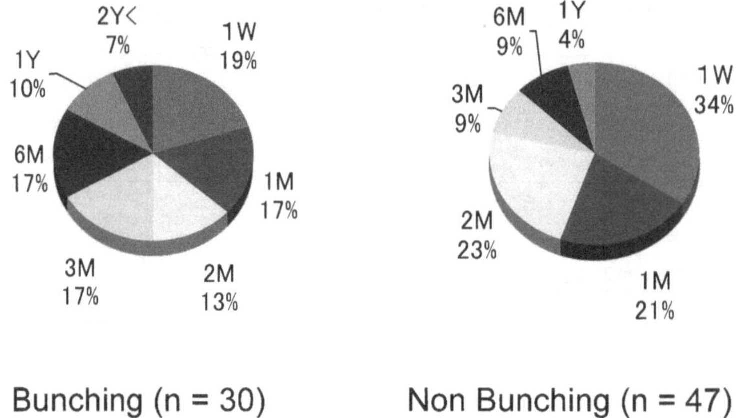

FIG. 4. Recovery of urinary continence in both DVC bunching and nonbunching subgroups of Group II

Functional Results

Recovery of urinary continence in both DVC bunching subgroup and DVC nonbunching subgroup of Group II are shown in Fig. 4. Thirty-six and 55% of the patients were almost dry (no pads in usual activity) at 1 month postoperatively in DVC bunching and DVC nonbunching groups, respectively. Sixty-six and 87% of the patients were almost dry at 3 months postoperatively in each group, respectively. Seven percent of the patients in the DVC bunching group still required more than one pad for stress incontinence at 2 years postoperatively.

Preservation of the unilateral neurovascular bundle was performed in 31 patients. Eight patients (25.8%) regained potency to be able to carry out sexual intercourse between 6 and 15 months. Two of the eight patients require sildenafil citrate.

Discussion

While the mean operating time of 356 ± 157 min in the first 30 cases had been decreased to 262 ± 60 min in the next 30 cases in Group I [4], that of the following Group II was still 291 ± 57.2 min. This seemed to be caused by modification of the procedure and establishment of new operating teams at the new institution. Guillonneau et al. also indicated that the mean operative time has been brought down to about 3 h after 300 cases experienced [6]. Fixation of the procedure and members of the operating team might be important factors. The blood transfusion rate in LRP was quite low (2%–5.7%) [7–10] except for the very initial experience (15.4% in 65 operations) by Guillonneau et al. [11].

In our experience blood transfusion including autologous blood was required only in the very early experience. By this reasoning, in recent experience autologous blood for transfusion is prepared only for the patients with a very high body mass index (BMI) to reduce cost.

Regarding technical aspects, several modifications appeared to be important in achieving less morbidity and better oncological and functional results. We introduced the balloon dissection method to enter the Retzius cavity after completing dissection of the seminal vesicle and vas deferens transperitoneally to avoid bladder injury [4]. We then tried a complete extraperitoneal approach in several cases including those patients with a high BMI. The procedure gave us a better view of the prevesical space without bowels and excessive fatty tissue; however, we noted a potential increase in traction on the vesicourethral anastomosis due to more limited bladder mobilization as indicated by Bollens et al. [12]. But our experience of the extraperitoneal approach is too small to agree with their opinion that there was no difference in the postoperative catheter indwelling period and continence recovery between extraperitoneal and transperitoneal approaches [12]. We also experienced difficulty in retrograde dissection of the seminal vesicle without using electrocautery for the nerve-sparing procedure. There are several reports that indicate no difference in PSM rates [13–15] and urinary continence recovery [14,15] between transperitoneal and extraperitoneal approaches; however, no reports reveal the equivalent result of recovery of erectile function in the extraperitoneal approach to that in the transperitoneal one. In this regard we returned to the original transperitoneal dissection of the seminal vesicle and the Retzius cavity with enough anatomical knowledge by experience to avoid bladder injury.

Positive surgical margins are one of the indices used to evaluate oncological results of radical prostatectomy in the early postoperative period, and it is a significant predictor of outcome for organ-confined disease (OCD) [16,17]. The rates of 13.8% for all pathological stages and 6.6% for OCD in our series are comparable to those in other LRP series (13.7% for all and 10.0% for OCD) [18]. Our data and those of Fromont et al. [18] are compatible to those in large cohort of RRP [19]. However, Fromont et al. indicated that a lower PSM rate at the apex in LRP as compared to RRP appeared to account for the lower PSM rates in LRP in their matched comparative study [18]. On the other hand Salomon et al. indicated a lower PSM rate at the bladder neck and higher posterolateral PSM rate in LRP compared with those of RRP and perineal radical prostatectomy [20]. A marked decrease of PSM at the bladder neck in our early experience seemed to be due to recognition of the correct plane of the prostate margin and improvement of dissection procedure through experience [4]. Our PSM rate of OCD itself (6.6%) was not so high; however, the apex was the most frequent PSM portion in our series (Fig. 5). Although Katz et al. recommended division of the puboprostatic ligaments to obtain a lower apical PSM [21], frequent modifications of the apical dissection procedure seems to be a likely cause of high apical PSM in our series. Too much attention toward protecting the urethral sphincter might cause inadequate apical dissection because there is no

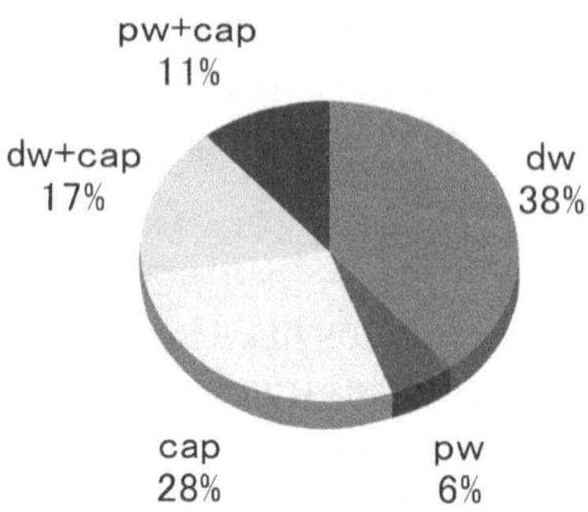

Fig. 5. Positive surgical margin sites

capsular structure at this portion. A video documentation review of intraoperative findings according to the pathology might be helpful in improving the procedure for quality assurance [22].

Urinary continence is the most important factor in postoperative quality of life (QOL) for radical prostatectomy. Many reports indicate that results of recovery of urinary continence in LRP (85.5%–90% at 1 year) [7,9,23] are close to those in recent RRP series (92%–93%) [24,25]. On the other hand, a more delayed recovery in the domain of urinary function and discomfort in health-related quality of life (HRQOL) after LRP than after RRP was reported when it was evaluated at 1 and 3 months postoperatively [26]. An apparent improvement in HRQOL was also indicated in the most recent LRP series when the LRP group was divided into two groups according to the surgical period [26]. To achieve more rapid recovery of urinary continence after LRP, we have made several technical modifications. The first one is the method of vesicourethral anastomosis. Although we had reported better water tightness in a single circumferential running suture for vesicourethral anastomosis [4], it seemed to be only a learning-curve effect in the subsequent experience. Our results had indicated no difference in continence recovery between eight interrupted sutures and a single circumferential running suture for vesicourethral anastomosis [4]. The second modification was a hemostatic procedure of DVC. We changed the procedure from a deep bunching of DVC to a vertical running suture of the cutting edge of DVC without DVC bunching to avoid ischemia of the urethral sphincter. After changing the DVC division procedure, we used interrupted sutures on the upper half of the urethra for anastomosis. It might be advantageous to pick up the shorter urethral edge with the DVC stump for anastomosis, leaving a longer urethral length proximal to the urethral sphincter. The third modification was preservation of the accessory pudendal vessels. This seems to be advantageous for preservation of the periurethral structure as well as blood supply to the urethra and the sphincter. After this change, the anastomotic procedure was also changed to nine interrupted sutures. The majority of patients after the third modification of apical dissection are not included in the DVC nonbunching group in Fig. 4; however, the DVC nonbunching group showed a more rapid recovery of urinary continence. When we looked at only the patients whose accessory pudendal vessels were preserved, they showed a trend toward more rapid recovery of urinary continence (data not shown).

Recovery rate of erectile function (25.8%) in our series was defined as the rate of postoperative feasibility of sexual intercourse. It was very approximate because the preoperative sexual function was not evaluated precisely. The patients analyzed had preserved unilateral NVB and the follow-up period was less than 2 years. While those patients with unilateral NVB preservation might require a longer postoperative period than those with bilateral NVB preservation (more than 50% at 6 months [8,23,27]), we expect that the recent procedure of pudendal vessel preservation might help earlier recovery of erectile function.

Conclusions

Operative morbidity control in LRP has been established in many institutions worldwide. Oncological control evaluated by PSM and early PSA recurrence rates after LRP are encouraging; however, long-term oncological results are required before LRP is firmly accepted as a tool for the treatment of organ-confined prostate cancer. While recovery of urinary continence 1 year after LRP appeared to be similar to that after RRP, a procedure to achieve more rapid recovery should be established to overcome the delay. The merit of a better, magnified view with less bleeding in LRP than in RRP must be reflected in the oncological and functional results following LRP.

References

1. Schuessler WW, Schulam PG, Clayman RV, Kavoussi LR (1997) Laparoscopic radical prostatectomy: initial short-term experience. Urology 50:854–857
2. Guillonneau B, Cathelineau X, Barret E, Rozet F, Vallancien G (1999) Laparoscopic radical prostatectomy: technical and early oncological assessment of 40 operations. Eur Urol 36:14–20
3. Trabulsi EJ, Guillonneau B (2005) Laparoscopic radical prostatectomy. J Urol 173: 1072–1079
4. Terachi T, Usui Y, Shima M, Okumura K (2004) Laparoscopic radical prostatectomy. In: Higashihara E, Naito S, Matsuda T (eds) Recent advances in endourology 5. Springer, Berlin Heidelberg New York Tokyo, pp 127–140
5. Guillonneau B, Vallancien G (2000) Laparoscopic radical prostatectomy: the Montsouris technique. J Urol 163:1643–1649
6. Guillonneau B, Rozet F, Cathelineau X, Lay F, Barret E, Doublet JD, Baumert H, Vallancien G (2002) Perioperative complications of laparoscopic radical prostatectomy: the Montsouris 3-year experience. J Urol 167:51–56
7. Hoznek A, Salomon L, Olsson LE, Antiphon P, Saint F, Cicco A, Chopin D, Abbou CC (2001) Laparoscopic radical prostatectomy. The Creteil experience. Eur Urol 40:38–45

8. Turk I, Deger S, Winkelmann B, Schonberger B, Loening SA (2001) Laparoscopic radical prostatectomy. Technical aspects and experience with 125 cases. Eur Urol 40:46–52
9. Eden CG, Cahill D, Vass JA, Adams TH, Dauleh MI (2002) Laparoscopic radical prostatectomy: the initial UK series. BJU Int 90:876–882
10. Dahl DM, L'Esperance JO, Trainer AF, Jiang Z, Gallagher K, Litwin DE, Blute RD Jr (2002) Laparoscopic radical prostatectomy: initial 70 cases at a U.S. university medical center. Urology 60:859–863
11. Guillonneau B, Vallancien G (1999) Laparoscopic radical prostatectomy: initial experience and preliminary assessment after 65 operations. Prostate 39:71–75
12. Bollens R, Vanden Bossche M, Roumeguere T, Damoun A, Ekane S, Hoffmann P, Zlotta AR, Schulman CC (2001) Extraperitoneal laparoscopic radical prostatectomy. Results after 50 cases. Eur Urol 40:65–69
13. Ruiz L, Salomon L, Hoznek A, Vordos D, Yiou R, de la Taille A, Abbou CC (2004) Comparison of early oncologic results of laparoscopic radical prostatectomy by extraperitoneal versus transperitoneal approach. Eur Urol 46:50–54
14. Erdogru T, Teber D, Frede T, Marrero R, Hammady A, Seemann O, Rassweiler J (2004) Comparison of transperitoneal and extraperitoneal laparoscopic radical prostatectomy using match-pair analysis. Eur Urol 46:312–319
15. Cathelineau X, Cahill D, Widmer H, Rozet F, Baumert H, Vallancien G (2004) Transperitoneal or extraperitoneal approach for laparoscopic radical prostatectomy: a false debate over a real challenge. J Urol 171:714–716
16. Ohori M, Wheeler TM, Kattan MW, Goto Y, Scardino PT (1995) Prognostic significance of positive surgical margins in radical prostatectomy specimens. J Urol 154:1818–1824
17. Guillonneau B, el-Fettouh H, Baumert H, Cathelineau X, Doublet JD, Fromont G, Vallancien G (2003) Laparoscopic radical prostatectomy: oncological evaluation after 1,000 cases at Montsouris Institute. J Urol 169:1261–1266
18. Fromont G, Guillonneau B, Validire P, Vallancien G (2002) Laparoscopic radical prostatectomy. Preliminary pathologic evaluation. Urology 60:661–665
19. Hull GW, Rabbani F, Abbas F, Wheeler TM, Kattan MW, Scardino PT (2002) Cancer control with radical prostatectomy alone in 1,000 consecutive patients. J Urol 167: 528–534
20. Salomon L, Anastasiadis AG, Levrel O, Katz R, Saint F, de la Taille A, Cicco A, Vordos D, Hoznek A, Chopin D, Abbou CC (2003) Location of positive surgical margins after retropubic, perineal, and laparoscopic radical prostatectomy for organ-confined prostate cancer. Urology 61:386–390
21. Katz R, Salomon L, Hoznek A, de la Taille A, Antiphon P, Abbou CC (2003) Positive surgical margins in laparoscopic radical prostatectomy: the impact of apical dissection, bladder neck remodeling and nerve preservation. J Urol 169:2049–2052
22. Touijer K, Kuroiwa K, Saranchuk JW, Hassen WA, Trabulsi EJ, Reuter VE, Guillonneau B (2005) Quality improvement in laparoscopic radical prostatectomy for pT2 prostate cancer: impact of video documentation review on positive surgical margin. J Urol 173:765–768
23. Guillonneau B, Cathelineau X, Doublet JD, Vallancien G (2001) Laparoscopic radical prostatectomy: the lessons learned. J Endourol 15:441–445
24. Catalona WJ, Carvalhal GF, Mager DE, Smith DS (1999) Potency, continence and complication rates in 1,870 consecutive radical retropubic prostatectomies. J Urol 162:433–438

25. Walsh PC, Marschke P, Ricker D, Burnett AL (2000) Patient-reported urinary continence and sexual function after anatomic radical prostatectomy. Urology 55:58–61
26. Namiki S, Egawa S, Baba S, Terachi T, Usui Y, Terai A, Tochigi T, Kuwahara M, Ioritani N, Arai Y (2005) Recovery of quality of life in year after laparoscopic or retropubic radical prostatectomy: a multi-institutional longitudinal study. Urology 65:517–523
27. Katz R, Salomon L, Hoznek A, de la Taille A, Vordos D, Cicco A, Chopin D, Abbou CC (2002) Patient reported sexual function following laparoscopic radical prostatectomy. J Urol 168:2078–2082

Laparoscopic Radical Prostatectomy: Extraperitoneal Approach

Ken Nakagawa and Masaru Murai

Summary. Many modifications of laparoscopic radical prostatectomy (LRP) have been tried and different methods of LRP have been established as the open retropubic radical prostatectomy. The initial dissection for vasa deferentia and seminal vesicles, which was an essential part of LRP as an established transperitoneal approach, has been unnecessary, and extraperitoneal LRP is now standardized and the steps of the procedure more clearly defined. Here, we highlight extraperitoneal LRP and the literature is reviewed. Extraperitoneal LRP has the valuable advantages of usual laparoscopic surgery and open retropubic radical prostatectomy. Laparoscopic surgery supplies less pain and reduces morbidity, leading to earlier recovery for the patients and a magnified, superior view for the surgeons. The extraperitoneal approach offers the elimination of possible risks, such as bowel injury, ileus, intraperitoneal bleeding and urine leakage, and allows possible later adjuvant radiation. Moreover, it may reduce the operating time and offers the same functioning and early oncological results as the transperitoneal approach. Lymphocele, which is a definite disadvantage of extraperitoneal LRP, should not become an issue because nomograms have reduced the necessity of its enforcement. Although a final answer may be decided only after long-term follow-up, extraperitoneal LRP should become one of our standard procedures.

Keywords. Laparoscopic radical prostatectomy, Extraperitoneal approach, Transperitoneal approach, Comparison of approaches for LRP, Advantages of extraperitoneal LRP

Department of Urology, Keio University School of Medicine, 35 Shinanomachi, Shinjuku-ku, Tokyo 160-8582, Japan

Introduction

Urological laparoscopic surgery has continued to spread dramatically for the last decade. It was initially applied to a diagnostic procedure as pelvic lymphadenectomy for prostate cancer [1,2], or only to resections as adrenalectomy [3] or nephrectomy [4]. Its use has expanded to reconstruction after resection, such as partial nephrectomy, radical cystectomy [5], and radical prostatectomy [6].

Although laparoscopic radical prostatectomy (LRP) was first described in 1992 by Schuessler et al. [7], their laparoscopic procedures could not define the obvious advantage to open radical prostatectomy. Groups in Bordeaux and Paris refined LRP and Guillonneau et al. [8] described their superior series as the Montsouris technique in 1998. It was a feasible transperitoneal approach, characterized by dissecting the vasa deferentia and seminal vesicles via the Douglas pouch at the beginning. Meanwhile, Raboy et al. [9] reported the first case of LRP with a purely extraperitoneal approach in 1997, and Bollens et al. [10] employed the extraperitoneal approach in their LRP series. The extraperitoneal approach is similar to open retropubic radical prostatectomy and avoids the complications related with intra-abdominal procedures. According to recent reports, the initial treatment of the vas deferens and seminal vesicles is an indispensable part of LRP, yet many groups are still using the Montsouris technique.

Extraperitoneal LRP is now standardized and the steps of the procedure are more clearly defined. In this chapter we highlight extraperitoneal LRP and the literature is reviewed. Also, our experiences of extraperitoneal LRP are described.

Surgical Technique of Extraperitoneal LRP [11]

In our institution, we started LRP using transperitoneal approach in 2000. After the experience of 30 cases using the transperitoneal approach (Fig. 1a) and 40 cases using the combined approach (Fig. 1b), including the transperitoneal approach for the Denonvilliers space via the Douglas pouch and the extraperitoneal approach for the Retzius space, we changed to the extraperitoneal approach as from 2002 (Fig. 1c). The extraperitoneal approach has been performed for 180 cases, and it is feasible and reproducible. We describe the details and technique.

Positioning and Instruments

Under general anesthesia, the patient is placed in the supine position and the arms are positioned along the body. The Trendelenburg position is not usually required. The surgeon stands to the left of the patient and an assistant and a camera-holder stand to the opposite side.

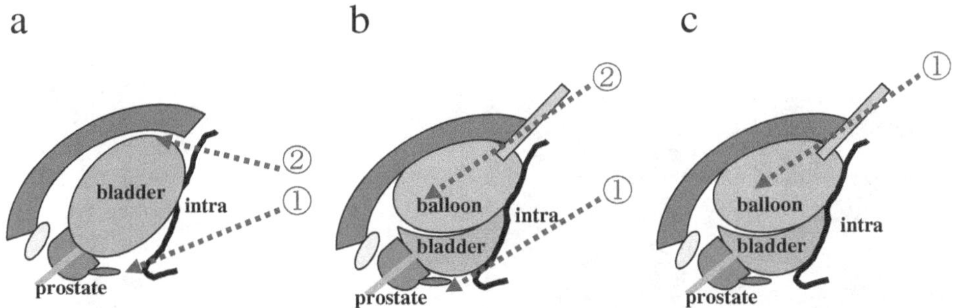

FIG. 1a–c. Surgical approaches for laparoscopic radical prostatectomy (LRP). **a** Transperitoneal approach. **b** Combined (transperitoneal+extraperitoneal) approach. **c** Extraperitoneal approach

The instruments are the same as with the transperitoneal approach, except for the balloon dilator. A suction and water pipe with a monopolar spatula and a bipolar forceps are very useful instruments, and are standard for the most manipulations in our laparoscopic surgery. Also, we prefer a flexible laparoscope both for transperitoneal and retroperitoneal LRP, as this is useful in the narrow Retzius space and reduces the time to exchange different angles of rigid scopes.

Placing Trocars

A 1.5-cm semicircumferential incision 1 cm below the umbilicus is used to access the extraperitoneal space. After blunt dissection to the anterior rectus fascia, the fascia is incised and the space between the rectus muscle and the posterior rectus sheath is made for a balloon dilator by finger dissection. Then the extraperitoneal space is developed with a balloon dilator. A 12-mm Hasson-type balloon trocar is placed into the space and CO_2 gas is inflated via the trocar at 12 mmHg. Once the extraperitoneal space has been developed, four trocars are inserted under laparoscopic view, as shown in Fig. 2. A 12-mm trocar is halfway from the umbilicus to the pubic symphysis. Two trocars (12 mm and 5 mm) are on the right side between the umbilicus and the ileum and a 5-mm trocar is on the left side. As the inferior epigastric vessels can always be identified in the extraperitoneal approach, the trocars are safely inserted for them.

Creation of the Working Space in Retzius Space and Pelvic Lymph Node Dissection

A bipolar forceps via the left trocar and a monopolar spatula via the suprapubic trocar are used for the additional extraperitoneal dissection. As the landmarks of the detached space, the following are exposed: longitudinally the pubic arch, the bladder, the prostate, the puboprostatic ligament, and the endopelvic

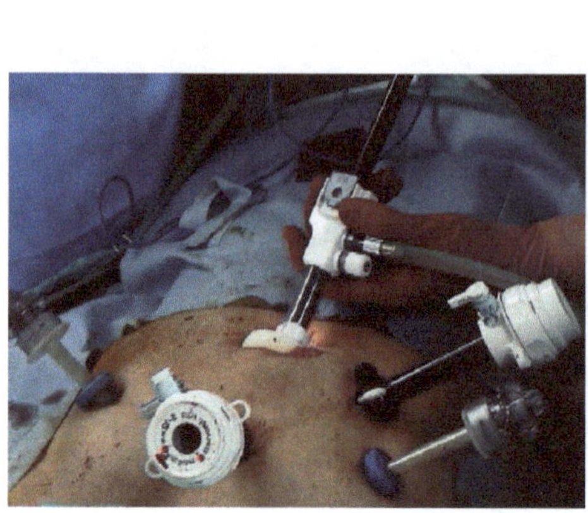

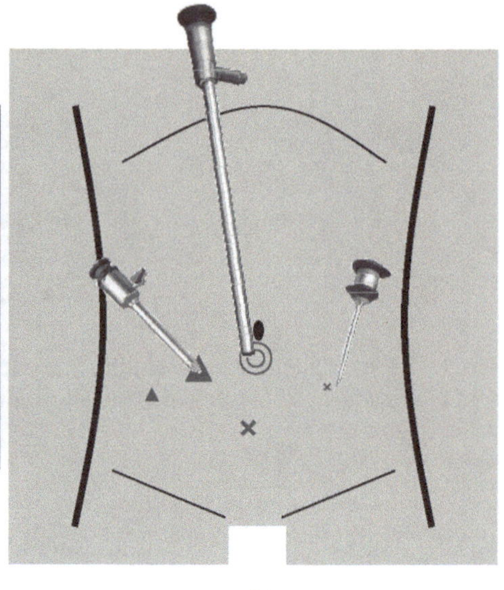

Fig. 2. Trocar position. *Concentric circles*, 12-mm Hassan-type trocar for laparoscope; *large cross*, 12-mm trocar for surgeon (*small cross*: 5 mm); *large triangle*, 12-mm trocar for assistant (*small triangle*: 5 mm)

fascia; laterally the obturator nerve, the external iliac vein, and the spermatic cord. The assistant helps to secure the working space with a retractor via a right 12-mm trocar. The fatty tissue is swept gently from the anterior surface of the prostate and the endopelvic fascia by suction. The superficial vein is treated with a bipolar forceps and transected.

Extraperitoneal pelvic lymph node dissection is an established laparoscopic procedure. The limits of the staging lymph node dissections at both sides are: cranially, the bifurcation of the common iliac artery; laterally, the iliac vein; medially, the medial umbilical ligament; caudally, the pubic bone; and posteriorly, the obturator nerve. But in our institute it has recently been omitted for those patients with a low prostate-specific antigen (PSA) level (<10 ng/ml) and low Gleason score (≤6) and limited lymph node dissection, which means just around the area of obturator nerve in the biopsy-positive side, is performed for the other patients. The blocks of the dissected lymph nodes are removed through the 12-mm suprapubic trocar.

Treatment of Apex

The endopelvic fascia is incised bilaterally. The prostate is retracted medially and the levator ani is detached to expose the pararectal fat laterally and apex medially. The vessels around the apex are treated with ultrasonic scissors, which min-

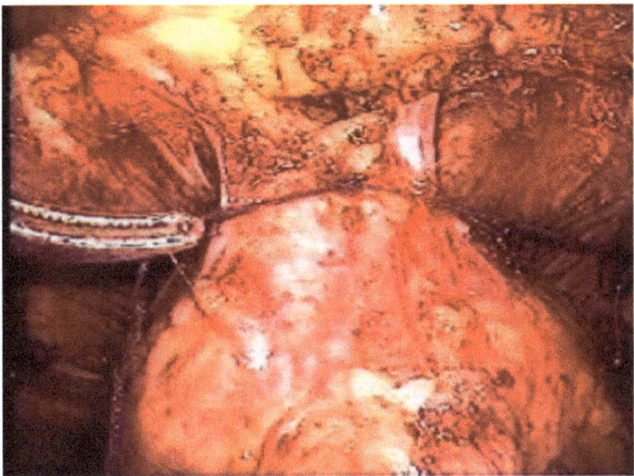

Fig. 3. Suturing of the dorsal vein complex behind the puboprostatic ligaments

imizes the heat damage to the neighboring tissue; an electric coagulation device is not used. The puboprostatic ligament is preserved to obtain the maximal stability of the urethra after the operation.

The dorsal vein complex (DVC) is clearly visible and is doubly ligated with a 2-0 absorbable suture (Polusorb™ 32 mm, 3/8 needle) behind the puboprostatic ligaments (Fig. 3). A proximal ligation of the DVC is not necessary.

Bladder Neck Dissection and Posterior Treatments

As the border between the prostate and the bladder can be identified by moving the urethral balloon catheter, the anterior bladder neck is divided in the midline. The dissection is continued laterally and deep until the urethra, peeling the bladder from the prostate, using the bipolar forceps and the monopolar spatula. The magnification of the laparoscope, which can recognize the muscle fiber of the bladder, easily identifies the plane, and the rinse and suction keep the operating field clear. After exposing the urethra as much as possible, the anterior wall of the urethra is incised and the deflated catheter is pulled up into the retropubic space. The assistant retracts the prostate ventrally using the catheter. After transecting the urethra completely, peeling of the bladder neck is continued to expose the vasa deferentia. The vasa deferentia are transected after treating with the bipolar forceps and the seminal vesicles are fully mobilized. When the nerve sparing is adopted, the dissection around the tips of the seminal vesicles should be done with care to avoid injury to the neurovascular bundles.

Incising Denonvilliers' Fascia and Sectioning of the Prostatic Lateral Pedicles

The assistant retracts the vasa deferentia and seminal vesicles ventrally and Denonvilliers' fascia is exposed. Denonvilliers' fascia is perforated horizontally from the midline and the prostate is bluntly dissected to the apex in the midline and laterally. The traction of the rectum to posterocranial direction is very important in order to avoid rectal injury. When nerve sparing is not adopted, the prostatic lateral pedicle is dissected with the ultrasonic scissors to the direction of the apex. The neurovascular bundle is separated sharply and bluntly with cold scissors for the nerve sparing. Bleeding from the neurovascular bundle after nerve sparing is usually controlled with careful astriction.

Apical Dissection and Extraction of the Prostate

Adjusting the angle of the forceps on the prostate, the DVC is cut carefully with the cold scissors from just at the front of the puboprostatic ligament. The laparoscopic magnified view supplies superior recognition of the cutting line, and the assistant rinses the area to keep it clear. After incising the anterior wall of the urethra, the urethral catheter is pulled up for the counter-traction. Then the remaining posterior wall and the rectourethralis are sharply divided. When nerve sparing is adopted, the neurovascular bundle is completely detached from the urethra before the posterior wall dissection. The freed prostate is placed in an endobag (Endo-Catch, Tyco) and is kept until completing hemostasis. Then the prostate is removed via the incision of the infraumbilical trocar. Depending on the size of the prostate, the skin incision is horizontally elongated to 3–4 cm and the fascia incision is longitudinally elongated. After removal, the elongated incision of the fascia is sutured for re-pneumocarbia.

Vesicourethral Anastomosis

A running vesicourethral anastomosis is performed with a 2-0 Polysorb™ (Tyco) suture on a 1/2 circle 27-mm needle. The running suture is started at 3 o'clock on the bladder and 7–9 sutures are usually performed. For the initial tying, the assistant lets the bladder come near to the urethra. The suprapubic trocar is used for the lateral sutures and the right trocar is used for the ventral and dorsal sutures. All sutures are placed outside-in at the bladder neck and inside-out at the urethra and Lapratie™ (Johnson & Johnson) after 4th and 6th sutures prevents loosening. When handling the urethra, a 16-F urethral bougie guides the suturing needle. A 20-F urethral balloon catheter is placed after the anastomosis and the water tightness is checked with saline. At the end of the procedure, a drainage tube is placed into the retropubic space through the 5-mm port-site in the left iliac fossa.

Clinical Experience of Extraperitoneal LRP in Keio University

We performed 180 cases of LRP using the extraperitoneal approach after the experience of an initial 30 cases using the transperitoneal approach and the next 40 cases using the combined approach. These changes of approaches were satisfactory and we have focused on the extraperitoneal approach described above.

Our patients were diagnosed as localized prostate cancer on computed tomography, bone scintigraphy, and transrectal magnetic resonance imaging. On average, patients were 65.9 years old (range 50–75 years old), had a mean PSA level of 11.2 ng/ml (4.1–52.6 ng/ml), a mean Gleason score of 5.8 (3–9), and an estimated prostate volume of 34.2 cm^3 (12–102 cm^3). In 180 extraperitoneal LRP procedures, the mean operative time was 198 min (106–407 min) and the mean blood loss including urine was 439 ml (0–4500 ml). All operations were completed laparoscopically but two patients (1.1%) needed blood transfusion and one (0.5%) experienced rectal injury. Also, 3 patients with lymphadenectomy (1.7%) needed drainage for their lymphoceles. The use of analgesics was 0.4 times (0–3 times) and all patients started walking on day 1. The average period of catheterizaton and postoperative hospitalization were 4.2 (3–17) and 6.3 (5–21) days, respectively. Recently, catheterization and postoperative hospitalization of almost all patients has been 3 days and 5 days, respectively. The positive surgical margin rate was 27% in all cases and 10% in pT2 cases. In the patients who have been followed for 1 year after their operations, PSA failure is 5.7%, and 97% of the patients do not have obvious incontinence.

Discussion of the Recent Knowledge on Extraperitoneal LRP

The first laparoscopic radical prostatectomy was performed by Schuessler et al. in 1991 [7] and French groups established reasonable procedures of LRP using the transperitoneal approach. Since then, LRP has been adopted worldwide, and LRP has shown lower morbidity and comparable oncological outcomes to the open procedure in the initial large series with a transperitoneal approach, known as the Montsouris technique [12]. Laparoscopic radical prostatectomy using the extraperitoneal approach was first described by Raboy et al. in 1997 [9] and Bollens et al. [10] followed this. Many modifications of LRP were tried, and different methods of LRP have been established as the open retropubic radical prostatectomy. Recently, four different approaches have been carried out: (1) transperitoneal descending prostatectomy with initial dissection of the vasa deferentia and seminal vesicles (Montsouris technique), (2) transperitoneal descending prostatectomy, (3) transperitoneal ascending prostatectomy, and (4) extraperitoneal descending prostatectomy. Transperitoneal descending prostatectomy and extraperitoneal descending prostatectomy are similar procedures, excepting treatment of the peritoneum.

We transferred to the extraperitoneal approach in 2002, because one case with vesical injury and several cases with severe adhesion of the digestive organs were experienced in our transperitoneal series. Urologists are familiar with the extraperitoneal approach by open retropubic radical prostatectomy. Extraperitoneal LRP has many considerable advantages. The extraperitoneal approach prevents the risk of intra-abdominal bowel injury and ileus. Several experiences of postoperative ileus, which needed surgical intervention, were reported from a Japanese institute. The extraperitoneal approach reduces injury of the epigastric vessels, which are recognized under the laparoscopic direct vision. As the preserved peritoneum serves as a natural bowel retractor, the operative field exposure is thereby facilitated and the degree of Trendelenburg position is reduced. Also, the extraperitoneal approach can be easily adopted for patients who had previous lower abdominal surgery (Fig. 4) but the transperitoneal approach is difficult for such patients. Another advantage is that, in the case of adjuvant radiotherapy, the bowel tract will not be in the radiation field. Finally, there may not be pain resulting from pneumoperitoneum.

Recently, the surgical outcomes of extraperitoneal LRP were compared with those of the transperitoneal approach. A French group reported that the elimination of the initial posterior dissection of seminal vesicles resulted in a significant shortening of extraperitoneal LRP operation time in comparison with the Montsouris procedure and extraperitoneal descending prostatectomy [13]. Direct access to Retzius' space can actually decrease operative time, especially for obese patients, because there is no time to dissect the bladder excessively. If there is bowel adhesion in the lower abdominal cavity, it would be much more obvious. When we started the extraperitoneal approach, the operating time was

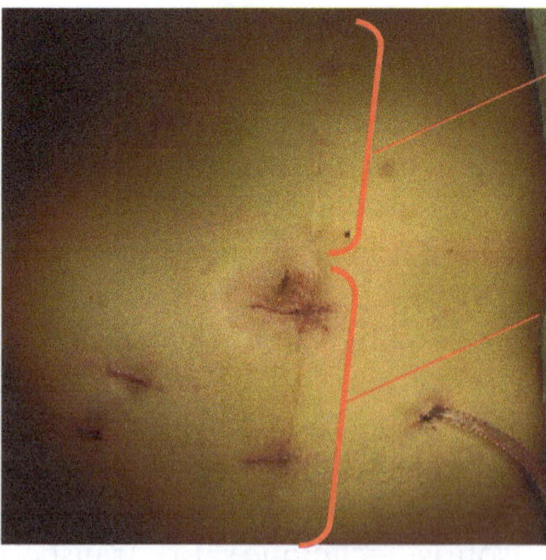

Fig. 4. Extraperitoneal LRP after previous abdominal surgery. Trocars were placed in the same positions as usual

reduced by 30 min compared with our previous transperitoneal procedures. But Erdogru et al. [14] insisted that the extraperitoneal approach did not reduce the operating time in their laparoscopic ascending prostatectomy series. This is a different result to other series and may be a feature of ascending prostatectomy (Table 1). In any case, the significant factor to reduce operating time in the extraperitoneal series may be the elimination of the initial posterior dissection. On the other hand, the rate of rectal injury was comparably low in both approaches. We experienced one case with rectal injury in each approach. Although the initial dissection of the seminal vesicles was the reason to choose the transperitoneal approach, it is no longer necessary. So there is no justification to continue using the transperitoneal approach regarding these points.

The most crucial factor in performing extraperitoneal LRP is whether it is able to reproduce the oncological results of transperitoneal LRP. The oncological results of transperitoneal LRP have been validated. Fromont et al. [15] and Salomon et al. [16] made pathological evaluations of their series of transperitoneal LRP and found that there was no difference in the risk of positive margins in comparison with their series of open retropubic radical prostatectomy. Guilloneau et al. [17] detailed comparable oncological results to open surgery in their large series of 1000 cases of transperitoneal LRP. Their positive surgical margins for pT2a, pT2b, pT3a, and pT3b were 6.9%, 18.6%, 30%, and 34%, respectively. Ruiz et al. [18] reported that the extraperitoneal approach offered the same early oncological results as the transperitoneal approach. The overall positive margin rates were 23% for the transperitoneal group and 29.7% for the extraperitoneal group ($P = 0.21$), and the positive margin rates of pT2 tumors were 13.0% and 17.0%, respectively ($P = 0.42$), despite the extraperitoneal group in their study having higher malignancy. Similarly, Erdogru et al. [14] did not find a significant difference when comparing the rate of positive surgical margins (overall 22.6% for the transperitoneal group vs 20.7% for the extraperitoneal group), neither for pT2 tumors (10% vs 7.3%) nor for pT3 tumors (61.5% vs 66.6%).

Surgeons who prefer transperitoneal LRP argue that the working space and the tension on the vesicourethral anastomosis are the disadvantages of extraperitoneal LRP. The whole space, especially around the umbilicus, of the transperitoneal approach is larger than that of the retroperitoneal approach. But the actual working space of LRP is the lower retropubic space, not around the umbilicus. The working space is limited by the pelvic bone structure but it is sufficiently large and similar to the transperitoneal approach. In our experience, daVinci with big shafts could work well in the space of the extraperitoneal approach. We logically understand the tension on the vesicourethral anastomosis in extraperitoneal LRP, because the extrapneumoperitoneum retracts the bladder cranially. But there was no trouble with suturing in our 180 cases of extraperitoneal LRP and the vesicourethral anastomosis in extraperitoneal LRP is not difficult in our opinion. According to the previous reports on extraperitoneal LRP, the vesicourethral anastomosis has no impact on the final results related to catheterization and continence (Table 1). Furthermore, we urologists

TABLE 1. Comparative issues between extraperitoneal and transperitoneal laparoscopic radical prostatectomy

	No. of patients	Operating time (min)	Transfusion (%)	Rectal injury (%)	Catheter (days)	Lymphocele (%)	Ileus (%)	Margin + (%; all/pT2)	Continence (%/12 months)
Our experience									
Extraperitoneal	180	198	1.1	0.5	4.2	1.7	—	27/10	97
Bollens et al. [10]									
Extraperitoneal	50	293	13	1.1	7.3	—	—	22/12.5	85
Stolzenburg et al. [19,21]									
Extraperitoneal	70/300	155	1.4	0.6	6.9	5.3	—	21.4/6.1	86
Guillonneau et al. [22]									
Transperitoneal	567	203	4.9	1.4	5.8	0.2	1	NA	NA
Cathelineau et al. [20]									
Transperitoneal	100	173	4	—	6.2	—	—	15/10	NA
Extraperitoneal	100	163	3	—	6.0	—	—	21/15	NA
Ruiz et al. [18]									
Transperitoneal	165	248	1.2	2.4	5.1	2.4	2.4	23/13	NA
Extraperitoneal	165	220	5.4	1.2	6.6	0.6	0.6	29.7/16.8	NA
Erdogru et al. [14]									
Transperitoneal	53	187	13	—	7	1.8	1.8	20.7/10	84.9
Extraperitoneal	53	191	16	1.8	7	—	—	22.6/7.3	86.7

NA, not available.

usually perform open retropubic radical prostatectomy extraperitoneally. There are enough anatomical landmarks in extraperitoneal LRP, unlike laparoscopic surgery with the extraperitoneal approach for the kidney or the adrenal.

The only real disadvantage of the extraperitoneal approach is lymphoceles. Stolzenburg et al. [19] reported postoperative lymphoceles in 5.7% of patients requiring percutaneous drainage in one third of their cases. In our series, 1.7% of the patients with simultaneous lymphadenectomy needed percutaneous drainage for their lymphoceles. In contrast, lymphoceles do not occur after the transperitoneal approach, because the lymphorrhea is diffused intra-abdominally and reabsorbed. But, under our indications for LRP, there is no lymph node metastasis in over 200 cases with lymphadenectomy and the indication of lymphadenectomy based on some nomograms has reduced the enforcement. Consequently, lymphoceles after extraperitoneal LRP should not become an issue.

The well-known institutes have mainly used the transperitoneal approach since the inception of LRP and they are much more familiar with it than extraperitoneal LRP. Under their situation, they have chosen the transperitoneal approach as from their comparative studies there was no big advantage apparent over the extraperitoneal approach. We agree that transperitoneal LRP is a valuable operation, but we think extraperitoneal LRP should become popular if the initial transperitoneal dissection for vasa deferentia and seminal vesicles is not necessary. If there is no difference both in the oncological and functional results, the possible risks to patients of the transperitoneal approach should be avoided. Also, the existence of the peritoneum as a retractor for the bowel is very agreeable for surgeons. Authors who previously reported preference for the transperitoneal approach have already acknowledged selective indications of the extraperitoneal approach for patients with obesity or previous abdominal surgery [14,22].

Conclusions (Table 2)

Pure extraperitoneal LRP has the valuable advantages of usual laparoscopic surgery and open retropubic radical prostatectomy. Laparoscopic surgery induces less pain, reduces morbidity, and aids earlier recovery for patients, and provides a magnified, superior view for surgeons. The extraperitoneal approach offers the elimination of possible risks, such as bowel injury, ileus, intraperitoneal bleeding, and urine leakage, and allows possible later adjuvant radiation. Also, it may reduce the operating time. A final answer will be decided upon after long-term follow-up because both transperitoneal and extraperitoneal LRP are still new procedures.

Table 2. Advantages and disadvantages of extraperitoneal laparoscopic radical prostatectomy

Advantages	No bowel injury No ileus Short operating time Easy for obesity Possible after previous lower abdominal surgery Prevents epigastric vessel injury Peritoneum as a natural retractor No Trendelenburg position No risk for adjuvant radiation Less pneumoperitoneum-related pain
No disadvantage	Positive surgical margin Catheterization Continence Rectal injury Working space
Disadvantages	Lymphocele Tension on anastomosis? (Whole space)

References

1. Schussler WW, Vancaillie TG, Reich H, Griffith DP (1991) Transperitoneal endo surgical lymphadenectomy in patients with localized prostate cancer. J Urol 145:988–991
2. Winfield HN, Donovan JF, See WA, Loening SA, Williams RD (1992) Laparoscopic pelvic lymph node dissection for genitourinary malignancies, indications, techniques, and results. J Endourol 6:103–109
3. Nakagawa K, Murai M, Deguchi N, Baba S, Tachibana M, Nakamura K, Tazaki H (1995) Laparoscopic adrenalectomy: clinical results in 25 patients. J Endourol 9:265–267
4. Baba S, Nakagawa K, Nakamura K, Deguchi N, Hata M, Murai M, Tazaki H (1996) Experience of 143 cases of laparoscopic surgery in urology. Clinical outcome in comparison to open surgery. Jpn J Urol 87:842–850
5. Nakagawa K (2003) Laparoscopic radical cystectomy. Urol View 1:79–85
6. Nakagawa K, Ohigashi T, Nakashima J, Marumo K, Murai M (2002) Laparoscopic radical prostatectomy: clinical results in 37 cases. Urol Surg 15:829–832
7. Schuessler WW, Shulam PG, Clayman RV, Kavoussi LR (1997) Laparoscopic radical prostatectomy: initial short term experience. Urology 50:854–857
8. Guillonneau B, Cathelineau X, Barret E, Rozet F, Vallancian G (1998) Prostatectomy radicale coelioscopique; premiere evaluation après 28 interventions. Presse Med 27:1570–1574
9. Raboy A, Ferzli G, Albert P (1997) Initial experience with extraperitoneal endoscopic radical retropubic prostatectomy. Urology 50:849–853
10. Bollens R, Vanden Bossche M, Roumeguere T, Damoun A, Ekane S, Hoffmann P, Zlotta AR, Schulmann CC (2001) Extraperitoneal laparoscopic radical prostatectomy. Results after 50 cases. Eur Urol 40:65–69

11. Nakagawa K (2005) Laparoscopic radical prostatectomy as a treatment for localized prostate cancer. Jpn J Endourol ESWL 18:58–63
12. Guillonneau B, Vallancian G (2000) Laparoscopic radical prostatectomy: the Montsouris experience. J Urol 163:418–422
13. Hoznek A, Antiphon P, Borkowski T, Gettman MT, Katz R, Salomon L, Zaki S, De La Taille A, Abbou CC (2003) Assessment of surgical technique and perioperative morbidity associated with extraperitoneal versus transperitoneal laparoscopic radical prostatectomy. Urology 61:617–622
14. Erdogru T, Teber D, Frede T, Marrero R, Hammady A, Seemann O, Rassweiler J (2004) Comparison of transperitoneal and extraperitoneal laparoscopic radical prostatectomy using match-pair analysis. Eur Urol 46:312–320
15. Fromont G, Guillonneau B, Validire P, Vallansian G (2002) Laparoscopic radical prostatectomy. Preliminary pathologic evaluation. Urology 60:661–665
16. Salomon L, Anastasiadis AG, Levrel O, Katz R, Saint F, de la Taille A, Cicco A, Vordos D, Hoznek A, Chopin D, Abbou CC (2003) Location of positive surgical margins after retropubic, perineal, and laparoscopic radical prostatectomy for organ-confined prostate cancer. Urology 61:386–390
17. Guillonneau B, El-Fettouh H, Baumert H, Cathelineau X, Doublet JD, Fromont G, Vallancien G (2003) Laparoscopic radical prostatectomy: oncological evaluation after 1000 cases at Montsouris institute. J Urol 169:1261–1266
18. Ruiz L, Salomon L, Hoznek A, Vordos D, Yiou R, de la Taille A, Abbou CC (2004) Comparison of early oncologic results of laparoscopic radical prostatectomy by extraperitoneal versus transperitoneal approach. Eur Urol 46:50–56
19. Stolzenburg JU, Do M, Rabenalt R, Pfeiffer H, Horn L, Truss MC, Jonas U, Dorschner W (2003) Endoscopic extraperitoneal radical prostatectomy: initial experience after 70 procedures. J Urol 169:2066–2071
20. Cathelineau X, Cahill D, Widmer H, Rozet F, Baumert H, Vallancien G (2004) Transperitoneal or extraperitoneal approach for laparoscopic radical prostatectomy: a false debate over a real challenge. J Urol 171:714–716
21. Stolzenburg JU, Truss MC, Rabenalt R, Do M, Pfeiffer H, Bekos A, Neuhaus J, Stief CG, Jonas U, Dorschner W (2004) Endoscopic extraperitoneal radical prostatectomy. Results after 300 procedures. Urologe A 43:698–707
22. Guillonneau B, Rozet F, Cathelineau X, Lay F, Barret E, Doublet JD, Baumert H, Vallancien G (2002) Perioperative complications of laparoscopic radical prostatectomy: the Montsouris 3-year experience. J Urol 167:51–56

Robotic Assisted Laparoscopic Radical Prostatectomy

MICHAEL J. FUMO, ASHOK K. HEMAL, and MANI MENON

Summary. Advances in robotics and laparoscopy have led to the advent of the union of their strengths to encourage laparoscopic reconstructive surgery. Radical prostatectomy has been the first procedure standardized and performed in large volume. This chapter will discuss the technique and evolution of robotic radical prostatectomy.

Keywords. Robotics, Robotic assisted laparoscopy, Prostatectomy

Introduction

Technological advances have always influenced and changed the way we live our daily lives. Advances in one field are quickly assimilated into another as potential uses are expanded upon to fill a void or improve upon a previous method. Medical science is very adept at adapting technological advances to its own needs in promoting patient care. Recent advances in robotics and audio-visual interfaces have been translated to medicine for the use of robotic assistance in surgery [1]. While surgery's ultimate goal, to cure patients of their disease state, has remained constant, the method of achieving that goal has evolved over time as the search continues for the most successful treatment with the least associated morbidity.

The discipline of surgery is currently undergoing a fundamental change in the method with which access to the organ of interest is approached. Common surgical thought states that exposure to the organ of interest is half the operation; inadequate surgical exposure can make a straightforward operation very difficult. Laparoscopy and minimally invasive procedures have gained acceptance and are quickly becoming the standard of care. Excellent surgical exposure

---

Vattikuti Urology Institute, Henry Ford Hospital, 2799 West Grand Boulevard, Detroit, MI 48202, USA

enhanced by magnification is available via laparoscopy, and at the same time multiple studies have proved time and again that patients have less perioperative pain and a quicker recuperation time after laparoscopic versus standard open procedures. Various urologic procedures have been retailored to a laparoscopic approach, the most difficult of which is laparoscopic radical prostatectomy. At one time this was considered impossible [2]; however, it has since been shown to be feasible and successful [3,4]. Robotics offers instruments that have a degree of precision and dexterity is unmatched even by the human hand [5]. The combination of the disciplines of laparoscopy and robotics, thus combining superior exposure with precise maneuverability, has offered the fulfillment of the potential of each while allowing widespread access to complicated reconstructive procedures in a laparoscopic, minimally invasive modality.

Robotic assisted laparoscopic radical prostatectomy is now standardized following the basic tenets of anatomic prostatectomy [6] and laparoscopic surgery [7]. Using the daVinci system (Intuitive Surgical, Mountain View, CA, USA) Menon et al. have now performed over 1500 cases of robotic radical prostatectomy (popularly known as the Vattikuti Institute Prostatectomy—VIP), the largest series in the world [5,8–10]. This chapter will discuss the technique of robotic radical prostatectomy using the daVinci robot, along with its advantages and disadvantages as the technique has evolved and been performed at the Vattikuti Urology Institute.

The Robot

The word "robot" is derived from the Czech word for forced labor or serf. The daVinci system follows in this definition in that the surgeon's console and surgical cart respectively follow the pattern of the master and slave relationship. The machine is designed with the goal of translating and refining the surgeon's movements into laparoscopic robotic movements. To this end the system comprises a surgeon's console, a surgical cart, and multiple interchangeable instruments.

The surgeons console is designed to display three-dimensional images in the orientation of open surgery through the use of the InSite Vision System, and to allow combinations of hand and foot controls to organize the machine's movements. The surgeon's fingertip movements are transposed to the tiny robotic instruments, while the foot pedals in combination with the hand controls command the camera and electrocautery. The movements have motion scaling and tremor elimination to maximize surgical precision.

The surgical arm cart is designed for maximal access to the patient with minimal effort. The robot has capabilities of having two or three instrument arms. For the purposes of prostatectomy we have found that only two are necessary. These instrument arms are designed for agile movement in real time with the surgeon's movements, have multiple positioning joints to easily access any patient anatomy, and offer quick release adaptors for instrument exchange. The single endoscope arm is designed to be steady, nontiring, and precise in movement to each position, thus offering a constant clear picture.

The instruments that the surgical cart uses are termed EndoWrist, thus describing their dynamic articulations that mimic the dexterity of the human wrist at the instrument tip. There are multiple tip designs for a wide range of procedures, and the instruments are designed for quick release to speed instrument changes intra-operatively.

Indications and Considerations

Robotic radical prostatectomy follows the tenets of open radical prostatectomy in the treatment of patients with localized carcinoma of prostate (T1, T2) based on their prostate-specific antigen (PSA), Gleason score, and digital rectal examination (DRE). Patients should be medically fit to undergo surgery especially with regard to operative position, as the steep Trendelenburg position with a thoracic wrap and relative dehydration intraoperatively may preclude patients with cardiac and pulmonary comorbidities from this approach. It is preferable that patients have a body mass index less than 30, and have had minimal previous abdominal surgeries; however, neither obesity nor previous abdominal surgeries need be a strict contraindication to this approach. The degree of difficulty of each procedure will be significantly increased as obesity can complicate access and often is a warning of significant pelvic fat stores that may mask anatomy. Previous surgeries with the possibility of numerous adhesions or a hostile abdomen warrant careful thought to consider the best approach. Many of our patients have had previous abdominal surgery including previous laparoscopic procedures; however, the basic tenets of laparoscopic access guide us. The need for a limited lysis of adhesions is commonplace after previous laparoscopic appendectomy, inguinal hernia repair, or cholecystectomy, yet not restrictive to the robotic portion if done correctly. The characteristic of the prostate must also be taken into account. Prostates that vary greatly from normal size in either a smaller or larger manner often will lack classic visual landmarks used during dissection. Large prostates, more than 100 g, will further complicate the procedure as angles of vision and approach of instruments can become too acute for comfortable access. A narrow pelvis can lead to the same difficulties with average-sized prostates. Other important considerations are a history of recurrent prostatitis, neoadjuvant hormonal therapy, or repeated prostatic biopsies, especially close to the time of surgery, as these factors can leave periprostatic tissue fibrosed, thus making the posterior dissection much more difficult. Overall, neither a previous history of surgery nor a complicated prostatic factor are contraindications to robotic radical prostatectomy; however, they do need to be taken into account in the operative planning.

Technique of Robotic Radical Prostatectomy

Preparation

Preoperatively the patient prepares for surgery by initiating a clear liquid diet 2 days before surgery followed by a mechanical oral or rectal bowel preparation the day before surgery. In the preoperative area, standard antibiotic prophylaxis is administered along with prophylactic antithrombotic therapy for which we prefer a subcutaneous injection of 5000 units of heparin. The risk of deep vein thrombosis (DVT) secondary to the factors of malignancy, pelvic surgery, prolonged immobilization, laparoscopy, and steep Trendelenburg positioning, we believe, requires some type of prophylaxis. Sequential compression devices are routinely placed during surgery as well. Lastly, a skin preparation per surgeon preference is optional.

Patient Positioning

General endotracheal anesthesia is mandated given the laparoscopic nature of the surgery as well as the patient's positioning. An orogastric tube is also placed during the procedure and removed at the time of extubation. The patient is placed in a supine, modified lithotomy position with his arms at the sides of his body to avoid the risk of brachial plexus injury. This will then be transferred to a steep Trendelenburg position. The patient should be supported via a thoracic wrap, which more comfortably supports the patient without placing undue pressure on the shoulders and causing postoperative pain. The legs are separated in flexion and abduction because the length of the robotic arms necessitates bringing the robotic stand-in between the legs. Care is taken to adequately pad the pressure points and lower extremities. The abdomen, genitalia, and upper thighs are prepped with an iodine-based preparation and draped. An 18-F Foley catheter is inserted in the sterile field, and the bladder is drained.

Placement of Laparoscopic Ports

Proper port placement is imperative for adequate robotic access to the pelvis. The VIP is a transperitoneal procedure, and port placement reflects this. An extraperitoneal approach may also be used to gain access to the prostate; however, great care must be maintained in port placement given the fact that in this circumstance the ports must be placed more caudal to avoid entering the peritoneal space. This therefore leads to a smaller working space with a greater likelihood of interaction between the instruments and the possibility of unrecognized bowel injuries if ports are not placed perfectly.

Three ports are required for the robotic arms and two to three ports for the assistants. Throughout our series we have performed surgeries employing a left and right assistant as part of our residency training process, thus necessitating three assistant ports; however, the procedure can just as easily be completed with only a right-side assistant. First, initial access to the peritoneum is gained with a Veress needle and then, after raising the initial intra-abdominal pressures to 20 mmHg for the placement of ports, the Veress needle is replaced with 12-mm trocar and a 30° laparoscope is inserted to transilluminate the abdominal wall. The rest of the ports are then placed under direct vision starting with the two 8-mm metal trocars for robotic arms which are placed 2–3 cm below the level of the umbilicus, lateral to the rectus muscle on either side. Next, a 12-mm trocar for passing needles, removing biopsy tissue material, and introducing clips, etc. is placed in the anterior axillary line, 3 cm above the right iliac crest for the right-side assistant. For each assistant a 5-mm trocar is placed between the camera port and the right-side robotic port while a second 5-mm trocar is then placed 4 cm superior to the left iliac crest along the left anterior axillary line. The daVinci robot is docked over the patient (Fig. 1). It is important to remember that the position of each trocar's insertion may vary from patient to patient as the anatomy of port placement varies based on height, weight, and previous operations. Great care must be taken to place the ports under direct vision, and any adhesions should be taken down to facilitate this. It is noteworthy that there are often physiologic adhesions in the left lower quadrant as well as around the cecum, and these adhesions should be released, first to allow proper port placement and secondly, to permit easy passage of assistant instruments into the pelvis thus avoiding unnecessary trauma to the bowels. The release of these pelvic adhesions will later aid in lymphadenectomy as well (Fig. 2).

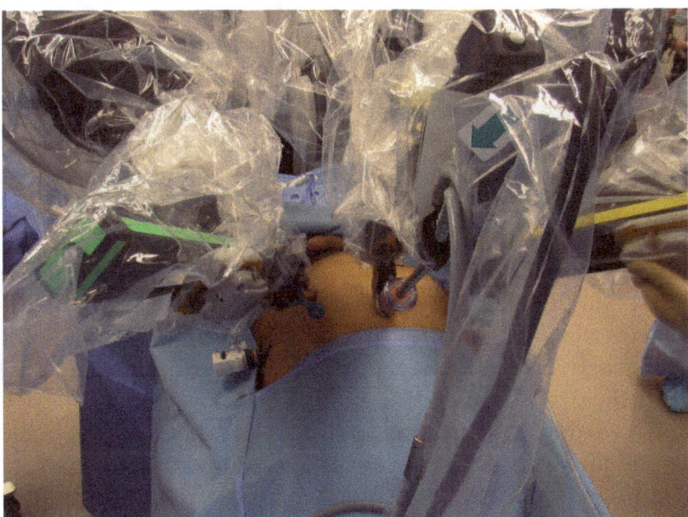

Fig. 1. General positioning in steep Trendelenburg position with legs in flexion. Note the placement of the ports and daVinci robot

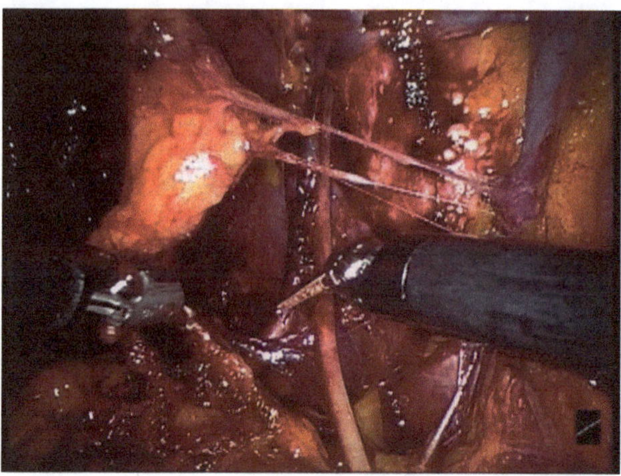

Fig. 2. Lymphadenectomy landmarks (external iliac vein, obturator nerve, and nodal packet) as posterior dissection is completed

Evolution of the Procedure

As in any procedure, there are modifications and additions as experience is gained and objective reviews of the results completed. The excellent visualization afforded by the endoscope allows the surgeon leeway to define exactly where the dissection will precede, thus affording varying degrees of preservation of tissues surrounding the neurovascular bundles depending upon the risk of extracapsular penetration as predicted by PSA, DRE, and biopsy results. Throughout the next steps of the procedure there will be comments with regard to how that step evolved with time.

Mobilization of Bladder

After all laparoscopic ports have been placed with dissection and removal of any adhesions, attention is then focused on entering the pre-peritoneal space. With the camera aimed 30° up, an inverted U-incision is made using the cautery hook so that the horizontal part of the incision is high enough on the anterior wall of the abdomen to preclude injury to the bladder and each vertical limb is located lateral to the medial umbilical ligament. This dissection is performed in the avascular plane involving the dissection of adipose and loose areolar tissue. The first landmark visualized is the pubic bone, and dissection is completed laterally on either side anteriorly, and completely exposing the endopelvic fascia bilaterally.

At this point the procedure may continue in one of two ways depending upon whether the endopelvic fascia will be spared. Recently, it has become our practice to offer patients with minimal cancer, as defined by low PSA, clinical T1C cancer, and minimal cancer detected on biopsy, with the option to have the endopelvic fascia spared in an attempt to dissect the prostate free with as minimal as possible interaction and trauma to the neurovascular bundles. In this circumstance the next two steps are skipped and dissection continues with the bladder neck transection with the endopelvic fascia still overlying the prostate. Otherwise the dissection continues with the apical dissection.

Apical Dissection

The endopelvic fascia is incised at the point where it reflects over the pelvic side wall, thus exposing the levator ani muscle which can then be gently dissected laterally to expose the lateral surfaces of the prostate. The incision is then extended toward the apex of the prostate to expose the dorsal vein, the urethra, and the striated urethral sphincter. The puboperinealis muscle covers the urethra and is the most anteromedial component of the levator ani; it has a special role in the urinary continence mechanism [11]. It is dissected bluntly from the apex of the prostate, thus exposing the urethra. The urethra should be dissected as little as possible and freed at the apex of the prostate from its underlying neurovascular bundles bilaterally, using only blunt dissection. Many small arterial and venous branches of the pudendal vessels are often encountered during this dissection and should be controlled with robotic bipolar forceps cautery.

Division of Puboprostatic Ligament and Control of Dorsal Venous Complex

Now that the anterior-lateral surfaces of the prostate and bladder are exposed, the camera is changed to a 0° lens. The fat over the prostate is then swept cephalad and laterally. In an effort to maximize continence, we routinely do not divide the puboprostatic ligaments, given that our exposure is excellent even with the ligaments intact [12]. A 0 vicryl suture on CT-1 needle is used to ligate the deep dorsal vein located behind the puboprostatic ligaments while attempting to exclude the puboprostatic ligaments (Fig. 3). Technically this is performed by passing the needle under the dorsal vein from one side to the other, and then it is grasped from the contralateral side, passed above the dorsal vein complex and under the puboprostatic ligaments. This way the ligaments are not included in the suture and thus the suture may be tied tighter.

Dissection and Division of the Bladder Neck

Moving forward with our dissection, we change over to a 30° angled lens directed downward for the bladder neck dissection. The identification of the bladder neck can be very difficult given that only vision can be depended on to find the junction. We employ multiple visual clues to find the proper plane of dissection. The movements of the inflated balloon inside the bladder may aid in demarcating the base of the prostate, and then the Foley catheter balloon is deflated. The bladder can now be grasped with a laparoscopic atraumatic grasper by an assistant and then retracted cephalad and to each side of dissection so as to identify the junction between the floppy bladder and the solid prostate. There is a shiny, smooth pad of fat that also helps to demarcate the prostatovesical junction. Start-

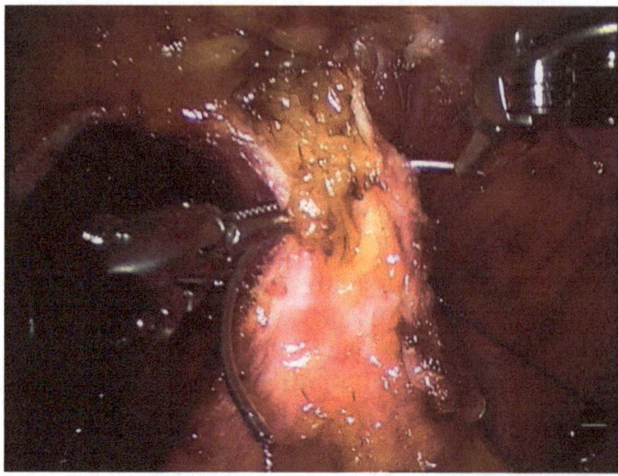

Fig. 3. Ligation of dorsal venous complex with preserved puboprostatic ligament

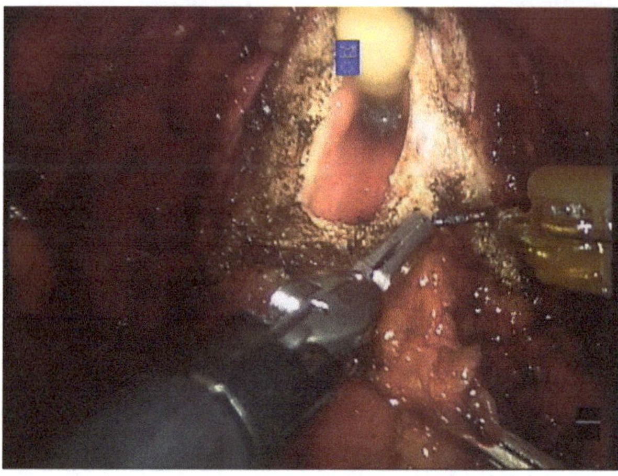

Fig. 4. Divided anterior bladder neck dissection with catheter retracted

ing laterally with a hook, gentle blunt dissection is employed to find the area where the shiny prevesical fat ends and to then make an incision there, which is then duplicated on the contralateral side, and finally both lateral incisions are then joined horizontally thus dividing the anterior bladder neck in the mid-line. As the dissection is carried down, the catheter should be encountered at which time the tip of the Foley catheter can be delivered through this opening (Fig. 4). The tip of the Foley catheter can then be grasped by an assistant and retracted upwards so as to help visualize rest of the dissection as the posterior wall of the bladder neck is divided. Great care must be taken at this point to localize and avoid the ureteral openings so as to avoid damage and to maintain a clear, wide detrusor margin for subsequent vesicourethral anastomosis. Larger prostate or prostates that have a large median lobe often distort the anatomy, which not only makes both the posterior and apical dissection difficult, but also may leave a large defect in the bladder that requires reconstruction prior to the vesicourethral anastomosis.

Posterior Dissection

The camera continues to be directed downward 30°. The previously made incision in the posterior bladder neck will lead to Denonvillier's fascia and is therefore followed down. An assistant grasps the tip of the Foley catheter and retracts it upward, thus exposing the space posterior to the prostate. Dissection is carried down until the ampulla of the vas deferens and seminal vesicles are encountered. The vas deferens should be divided before commencing with the dissection of the seminal vesicles. The seminal vesicles are dissected using both blunt and sharp skills with the aid of retraction from the assistants. One must be mindful about the artery to the vas, which passes between the vas and the seminal vesicle and requires control before the seminal vesicle can be fully dissected free to its base. Attempts should be made to use minimal electrocautery so as to avoid heat or electrical injury to the neurovascular bundles. Both seminal vesicles are freed circumferentially. The seminal vesicles and vas are now used as a leverage point to retract the entire prostate upwards thus exposing the prostatic pedicles. The pedicles are well vascularized, and can be controlled prior to their division with two clips or with bipolar forceps and round-tipped robotic scissors. Lastly, the seminal vesicles are lifted up anteriorly to demonstrate the longitudinal fibers of Denonvillier's fascia near the apex of the prostate so that a transverse incision can be made deep enough to appreciate the prerectal fat posteriorly, thus completing the posterior dissection.

Nerve Sparing

The camera continues to be directed downward 30° while the robotic arms are left as articulated scissors and bipolar forceps. The packet of tissue containing the neurovascular bundles is freed, starting by incising the lateral pelvic fascia anteriomedially and parallel to the neurovascular bundles between the prostatic venous plexus and the prostatic capsule. The posterolateral surface of the prostate is sharply cleared by dropping a layer of fascia, fat, nerves, and blood vessels from the base and working toward the apex. Most of the dissection occurs in a relatively avascular plane, such that the neurovascular bundles can be freed from the prostate laterally and easily without the use of cautery. If needed, bipolar cautery alone can be used to control dissected, isolated vessels. The neurovascular bundles should now be completely freed of the prostate since each step in the dissection has been optimized in light of nerve preservation.

As the development of our approach has evolved, we have made some important technical modifications. One of the most important is an attempt to spare the accessory penile and cavernosal nerves which may course along the side of

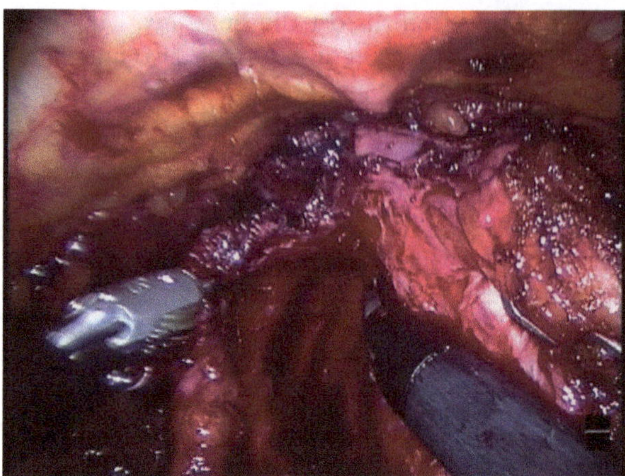

Fig. 5. View after completed apical dissection posteriorly and preserved left Veil of Aphrodite (nerve sparing)

the prostate. Animal and human studies suggest that there may be accessory cavernosal nerves that run underneath the lateral pelvic fascia on the anterolateral surface of the prostate [13]. These nerves may be physiologically relevant in erectile function. Given the improved vision and robotic manipulation, it is feasible to dissect this lateral fascia free of the prostate. In young patients without significant risk for extraprostatic extension, the lateral periprostatic fascia is preserved, creating a veil of tissue, the "Veil of Aphrodite" (Fig. 5).

In attempts to further improve the nerve-sparing dissection the endopelvic fascia may be spared in patients with low volume disease, as previously mentioned. The apical dissection and dorsal venous complex have not been dissected nor controlled in this case. Once again after the posterior dissection is completed the endopelvic fascia is incised parallel to the neurovascular bundles, with the goal of entering the lateral pelvic fascia anteromedially and parallel to the neurovascular bundles between the prostatic venous plexus and the prostatic capsule carried all the way distally to the apex. With this method all the tissues lateral and posterolateral to the prostate are left as undisturbed as possible.

Division of the Urethra

The urethra should now be the last connection remaining to the prostate. At this point the camera is changed to a 0° lens. Once again the long ends of the previously placed anterior deep dorsal vein sutures are grasped and retracted cephalad so as to stretch the urethra and dorsal vein complex, thus making them prominent and taut. The previously ligated dorsal venous complex is now divided with scissors proximal to the puboprostatic ligaments, and the incision is continued to divide the urethra at the apex of the prostate. Great care is taken to preserve as much urethral stump as possible to facilitate anastomosis. With the anterior urethral wall divided, the catheter is retracted out and care is taken to

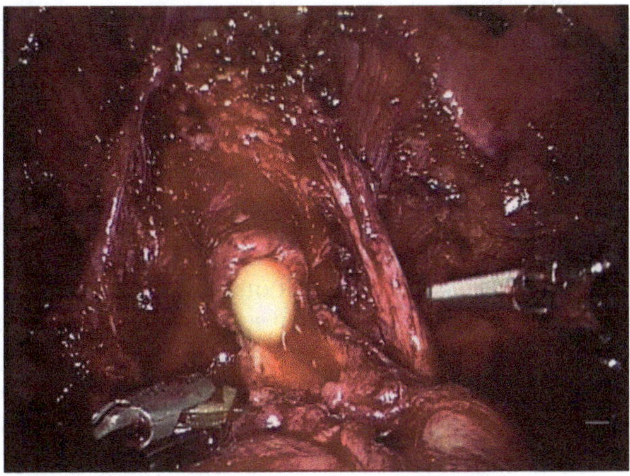

FIG. 6. Urethral transection with preserved neurovascular bundle (bilateral Veil of Aphrodite)

ensure that the neurovascular bundles have been freed laterally such that the last remaining tissue, posterior urethral wall, and the rectourethralis muscle can be sharply incised (Fig. 6).

Parietal Biopsies

Given the constraints of the anatomic dissection, we believe in biopsies at the margins. Parietal biopsies from the anterior, posterior, and lateral margins of the urethra as well as from the bladder neck are sharply excised and sent for frozen section. Depending upon the results of the biopsies, the margins are further resected as appropriate.

Lymphadenectomy

Bilateral pelvic lymphadenectomy is performed in standard fashion. This step is performed with a 0° and occasionally a 30° lens directed downward for proximal dissection, especially at the bifurcation of common iliac vessel. The internal inguinal ring can easily be seen, and laterally the external iliac vessels are hidden in a lateral fold of the peritoneum. The peritoneal incision is extended posteriorly as far as needed, now lateral to the medial umbilical ligament and medial and inferior to the internal inguinal ring. The nodal package will be lifted off the anterior surface of the external iliac vessels medially. Starting at the medial border of the external iliac vein, the nodal packet is cleaned medially, and careful dissection continues along its inferior border until the obturator nerve is identified (Fig. 2). The obturator nerve serves as the inferior margin of dissection. This nodal package contains the external iliac and the obturator nodes. Each nodal package and the prostate are now placed into a 10-mm Endocatch specimen bag (US Surgical, Norwalk, CT, USA), and the bag is then placed in the left upper quadrant of the abdomen until the end of the procedure.

Vesicourethral Anastomosis

The vesicourethral anastomosis has evolved over the course of our experience. Initially it was performed with eight interrupted sutures; however, we have currently advanced to a continuous anastomosis [14]. The tails of two 3-0 poliglecaprone 25 (monofilament) sutures (one dyed and one undyed for ease of identification during anastomosis) on an RB-1 needle (Ethicon, USA) are tied together extracorporeally. The total length of the suture varies according to the diameter of the bladder neck, and it may be anywhere from 12 to 18 cm as required. Bladder neck reconstruction is routinely carried out as needed with 2-0 vicryl using lateral sutures to decrease the size of the bladder neck. The final suture for anastomosis has a knot in the center and needles at either end of a dyed and an undyed suture. A 0° laparoscopic lens is employed with a left-handed Endowrist long-tip forceps and a right-handed Endowrist large-needle driver. The anastomosis is begun by passing the needle outside in at the 4 or 5 o'clock position on the bladder neck and inside-out on the urethra. After two or three throws on the urethra and three to four throws on the bladder to create an adequate posterior base, the suture is doubly locked and bladder is cinched down against the knot of the sutures lying on the posterior surface of the bladder. At this point, the long tip forceps is replaced with the large needle driver and the anastomosis is continued clockwise to the 9 o'clock position on the bladder. The suture is then turned into the bladder in such a way that it runs inside-out on the bladder and outside-in on the urethra to continue further up to the 11 or 12 o'clock position. Then the suture (dyed) is pulled cephalad toward the left lateral side of the pelvis and maintained under traction by an assistant. Subsequently, the anastomosis is started on the right side of the urethra with the undyed end, passing it outside-in on the urethra and then inside-out on the bladder, from the point where the anastomosis was started and continuing counterclockwise to the point where the other suture is met. After the initial two throws with the undyed suture, it too is also doubly locked as previously performed with the dyed suture. The needle of the dyed end is cut off, and the free dyed end and undyed ends are tied together with several knots (Figs. 7 and 8). The urethral catheter is used throughout the anastomosis as a guide in showing the urethral mucosa and finally is advanced into the bladder just before tying the sutures. The patency of the urethrovesical anastomosis is tested via instillation of 150–200 ml of water. If no leakage is seen the balloon of the Foley catheter is inflated. Sometimes bladder neck reconstruction is not deemed as necessary prior to the anastomosis, but if after completing the urethrovesical anastomosis there remains a large opening, the bladder neck can then be refashioned with interrupted full thickness sutures of 3-0 absorbable sutures.

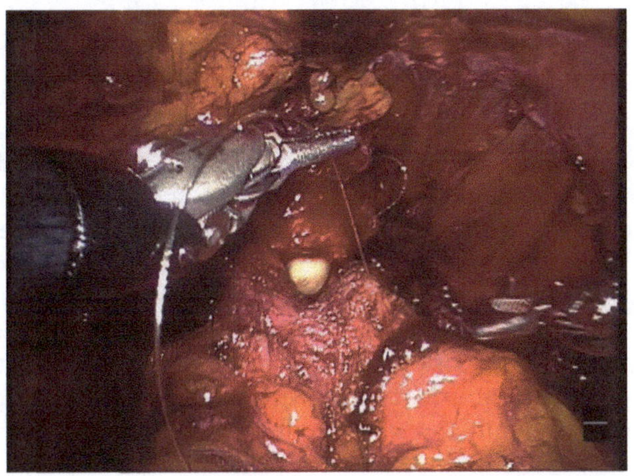

Fig. 7. Urethrovesical anastomosis in progress

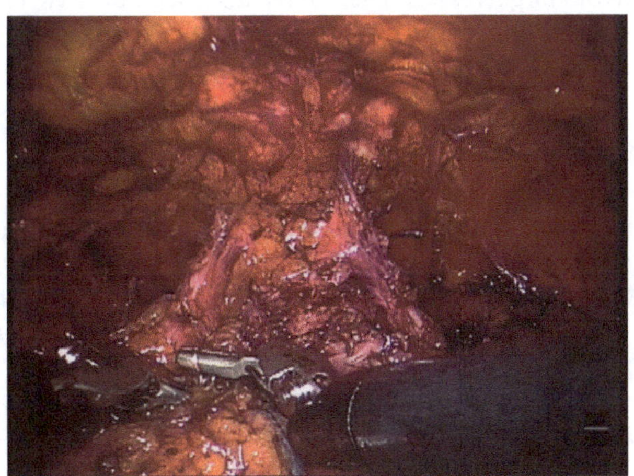

Fig. 8. Completed urethrovesical anastomosis

Retrieval of Specimen and Closure of Ports

The specimen is extracted via the umbilical port with extension of the semicircular incision as needed. Fascial closure is performed only at this incision given its size. Since small noncutting trocars are used for all ports except the umbilical site, these other ports are closed with subcuticular skin sutures only. A Jackson–Pratt drain is left extending into the pelvis from one of the 5-mm ports.

Complications

Robotic radical prostatectomy has offered excellent results with minimal morbidity. There have not been any intraoperative complications or conversions to an open approach, and no patient has required intraoperative transfusion. Minimal venous thrombosis has been observed during our series, probably as a result of excellent perioperative prophylaxis and also due to the fact that the transperitoneal approach makes lymphocele unlikely with secondary venous thrombosis unlikely as well. Unfortunately, the transperitoneal approach places the peritoneum in continuum with the urethrovesical anastomosis, which leaves the bowels at risk for irritation and ileus secondary to anastomotic leak. In cases of significant urinary leak with fluid collection, the patients present with significant abdominal distention and pain. Foley catheter drainage is the first step in treatment; however, there has been a need for postoperative computed tomography-guided drain placement to remove urine from the peritoneum until healing of the anastomosis is complete. There have been minimal port site hematomas as the ports are placed under transillumination in an attempt to avoid large vessels. There have also been only two port site hernias in over 1000 cases requiring surgical repair, despite the fact that we routinely close only the fascia of the umbilical port.

Results

Outcomes after robotic assisted laparoscopic radical prostatectomy are very impressive. The vast majority of patients are discharged from the hospital within 24h of surgery. Patients are discharged with a urethral catheter in place, which is usually removed within 7–10 days of surgery. Intraoperative blood loss averages around 150ml, and operative time averages around 140min. Long-term complications of urinary incontinence and impotence are minimized as well. Our patients have vastly better urinary control, which returns more rapidly, and improved potency as compared with open radical retropubic prostatectomy performed at our institution [15].

Conclusions

Technology has irreversibly changed the face of surgery. Surgical management continues to rest on the foundation of a sound knowledge of anatomy and physiology. However, there now exist tools to help expose anatomy better than has been normally seen, thus allowing precise surgical dissection to protect the physiology of the continence and erectile function in males undergoing radical prostatectomy. Robotics goes further in its superiority in the more facile performance of complex reconstructive maneuvers such as urethrovesical anastomosis. This has allowed for improved patient outcomes with a minimum of morbidity and improved patient satisfaction. Robotics offers the next natural advancement of laparoscopic surgery, as made evident by the great success of robotic radical prostatectomy, and now awaits further application to other disease processes [16–18].

References

1. Abbou CC, Hoznek A, Salomon L, Olsson LE, Lobontiu A, Saint F, Cicco A, Antiphon P, Chopin D (2001) Laparoscopic radical prostatectomy with a remote controlled robot. J Urol 166:1964–1966
2. Schuessler WW, Schulam PG, Clayman RV, et al (1997) Laparoscopic radical prostatectomy: initial short term experience. Urology 50:854–857
3. Abbou CC, Salomon A, Hoznek A, et al (2000) Laparoscopic radical prostatectomy: preliminary results. Urology 55:630–634
4. Guillonneau B, Vallancien G (2000) Laparoscopic radical prostatectomy: the Montsouris experience. J Urol 163:418–422
5. Tewari A, Peabody J, Sarle R, Balakrishnan G, Hemal AK, Shrivastava A, Menon M (2002) Technique of daVinci Robot-assisted anatomic radical prostatectomy. Urology 60:569–572
6. Walsh PC (1998) Anatomic radical prostatectomy: evolution of the surgical technique. J Urol 160:2418–2124
7. Gill IS, Kerbl K, Meraney AM, Clayman RV (2002) Basic principles, techniques, and equipment of laparoscopic surgery. Campbell's urology, 8th edn. Saunders, New York, pp 3455–3505
8. Menon M, Tewari A, Peabody JO, Shrivastava A, Kaul S, Bhanclari A, Hemal AK. Vattikuti Institute Prostatectomy, a technique of Mobotic Radical prostatectomy for management of localized carcinorma of the prostate: experience of over 1100 cases. Urol Clin North AM 2004 Nov; 31(4):701–717.
9. Menon M, Shrivastava A, Tewari A, Sarle R, Hemal A, Peabody JO, Vallancien G (2002) Laparoscopic and robot assisted radical prostatectomy: establishment of a structured program and preliminary analysis of outcomes. J Urol 168(3):945–949
10. Menon M, Tewari A, Peabody J, the VIP Team (2003) Vattikuti Institute prostatectomy: technique. J Urol 169:2289–2292
11. Steiner MS (1994) The puboprostatic ligament and the male urethral suspensory mechanism: an anatomic study. Urology 44:530–534
12. Deliveliotis C, Protogerou V, Alargof E, et al (2002) Radical prostatectomy. Bladder neck preservation and puboprostatic ligament sparing—effects on continence and positive margins. Urology 60:855–858
13. Tewari A, Peabody JO, Fischer M, Sarle R, Vallancien G, Delmas V, Hassan M, Bansal A, Hemal AK, Guillonneau B, Menon M (2003) An operative and anatomic study to help in nerve sparing during laparoscopic and robotic radical prostatectomy. Eur Urol 43(5):444–454
14. Menon M, Hemal AK, Tewari A, Shrivastava A, Bhandari A (2004) The technique of apical dissection of the prostate and urethrovesical anastomosis in robotic radical prostatectomy. BJU Int 93(6):715–719
15. Tewari A, Shrivastava A, Menon M, et al (2003) A prospective comparison of radical retropubic and robot-assisted prostatectomy: experience in one institution. BJU Int 92(3):205–210

16. Hemal AK, Menon M (2004) Robotics in urology. Curr Opin Urol 14(2):89–94
17. Menon M, Hemal AK, Tewari A, Shrivastava A, Shoma A, Ghoneim MA (2004) Robot-assisted radical cystectomy and urinary diversion in female patients: technique with preservation of the uterus and vagina. J Am Coll Surg 198(3):386–393
18. Menon M, Hemal AK, Tewari A, Shrivastava A, Shoma AM, El-Tabey NA, Shaaban A, Abol-Enein H, Ghoneim MA (2003) Nerve-sparing robot-assisted radical cystoprostatectomy and urinary diversion. BJU Int 92(3):232–236

Part 5
Testis: Retroperitoneal Lymph Node

Laparoscopic Retroperitoneal Lymph Node Dissection: Transperitoneal Approach

NASSER ALBQAMI and GÜNTER JANETSCHEK

Summary. To lower the morbidity of retroperitoneal lymphadenectomy, the procedure was modified over the past 35 years from extended suprahilar to bilateral infrahilar, and subsequently a modified laparoscopic unilateral approach then a nerve-sparing technique was introduced. There was no increase in relapse rates associated with the introduction of these operative refinements; significant factors for relapse were pathological stage ($P < 0.001$) and adjuvant chemotherapy in stage II disease ($P < 0.001$) [8]. Laparoscopic retroperitoneal lymph node dissection (RPLND) has been advocated and utilized in the management of testicular cancer over the past decade. This method technically duplicates the open surgical technique and has demonstrated its surgical and oncologic efficacy. The morbidity and complication rates are low. Tumor recurrence rates after laparoscopic RPLND are comparable to those of open surgery. Laparoscopic RPLND is safe, with less postoperative morbidity, quicker convalescence, improved cosmetic results, and a diagnostic accuracy equal to that of the open technique.

Keywords. Testicular cancer, Retroperitoneal lymph node dissection, Laparoscopy, Transperitoneal approach, Chemotherapy

Introduction

Testicular cancer is the most common malignancy in men between 15 and 35 years of age. Clinical staging is the first step in the management of all testicular cancer patients after radical orchiectomy. Retroperitoneal lymphadenectomy is the most sensitive and specific method for testicular cancer staging.

Currently, testicular tumors show excellent cure rates. The main factors contributing to this are careful staging at the time of diagnosis, adequate early treat-

Department of Urology, Elisabethinen Hospital, Postfach 239, Fadingerstrasse 1, 4010 Linz, Austria

ment based on chemotherapeutic combinations with or without radiotherapy and surgery, and very strict follow-up and salvage therapies.

In clinical stage I nonseminomatous germ cell tumors (NSGCT) high cure rates can be achieved by three therapeutic strategies: retroperitoneal lymph node dissection (RPLND), surveillance, and risk adapted therapy including surveillance for low-risk patients and adjuvant chemotherapy for high-risk groups. RPLND is still the preferred treatment of choice in many institutes for stage I NSGCT because of the added advantage of correct staging and the immediate stratification for further treatment options, i.e., adjuvant chemotherapy or surveillance. We have replaced the open surgical technique by laparoscopy since laparoscopic RPLND technically duplicates the open surgical technique and has been proven to be safe, with less postoperative morbidity, quicker convalescence, improved cosmetic results, and a diagnostic accuracy equal that of the open technique [1–4].

Patients clinically diagnosed as stage II NSGCT are treated classically by either primary chemotherapy (3–4 cycles) followed by RPLND if residual retroperitoneal masses are observed or by open RPLND without or with adjuvant chemotherapy. We adhered to the concept of primary chemotherapy for this stage, but we attempted to reduce its morbidity while maintaining its oncologic efficiency. It would be ideal to give the minimum dose required for complete tumor response and to avoid any overdose which would only add morbidity without any therapeutic effect. To achieve this goal we reduced the dose of chemotherapy to two cycles of bleomycin, etoposide, and cisplatin (BEP) in stage IIB patients (2–5 cm retroperitoneal tumors). However, to control the complete response, RPLND becomes mandatory even if there is no residual tumor. Again to reduce the morbidity of open RPLND, it was replaced by laparoscopy and in our experience, morbidity of postchemotherapy laparoscopic RPLND is clearly less than that of a third or even a fourth cycle of chemotherapy.

Contraindications for Laparoscopic RPLND

The absolute contraindications are elevated tumor markers, severe pulmonary fibrosis that prevents pneumoperitoneum, and uncontrolled bleeding diathesis. Patients with a higher body mass index benefit more from laparoscopy than slim patients with respect to postoperative pain and morbidity but do not experience more complications [5].

Preoperative Preparations

One day preoperatively, oral mechanical bowel preparation including clear fluid diet and laxatives is performed. All patients receive low-dose systemic antibiotic coverage on the day of surgery. Typing and cross-matching are performed for two units of blood. Preoperative preparations now include a low-fat diet for 1 week that is continued 2 weeks postoperatively as a measure to prevent chylous ascites, which was observed in some patients after postchemotherapy laparoscopic RPLND. The authors have not seen this complication since use of this precaution was instigated. A normal level of tumor markers is a prerequisite for RPLND.

Technique

Standard laparoscopic equipment used includes a three-chip video camera and a 30° laparoscope. The laparoscope is held and maneuvered by a robotic arm (computer motion, Santa Barbara, CA, USA). This has the advantage of providing stable video images even during lengthy procedures. Insufflation with a high flow rate has proved helpful because it prevents the pneumoperitoneum from collapsing during suction. All dissection is performed using bipolar grasping forceps and monopolar scissors. A small surgical sponge held with an atraumatic grasper is used for retraction, dissection, and hemostasis. A right-angled dissector (Aesculap, Germany) is applied for dissection of the vessels. We no longer use metallic clips but have replaced them with Hem-o-lok clips (Weck Closure Systems, Research Triangle Park, NC, USA).

Templates

Weissbach and Boedefeld have described templates that included practically all primary landing sites of lymph node metastases for patients diagnosed having NSGCT clinical stage I [6]. The right template will hold 97%, while the left template will hold 95% of all the primary landing sites of lymph node metastases in this stage.

The right template includes the interaortocaval lymph nodes, preoartic tissue between the left renal vein and the inferior mesenteric artery, precaval tissue, and all the tissues lateral to the vena cava and the right common iliac artery, while the lateral border of dissection is the ureter. The left template includes preoartic tissue between the left renal vein and the inferior mesenteric artery, all the tissue lateral to the aorta and the left common iliac artery and the interaortocaval lymph nodes, while the lymphatic tissue ventral to the aorta below the inferior mesenteric artery is preserved. The lateral border of dissection is the ureter (Fig. 1).

Procedure

The patient is placed with the ipsilateral side elevated 45° off the operating table. The operating table is then slightly flexed at the umbilicus. A Veress needle is used for the initial stab incision at the umbilicus to create the pneumoperi-

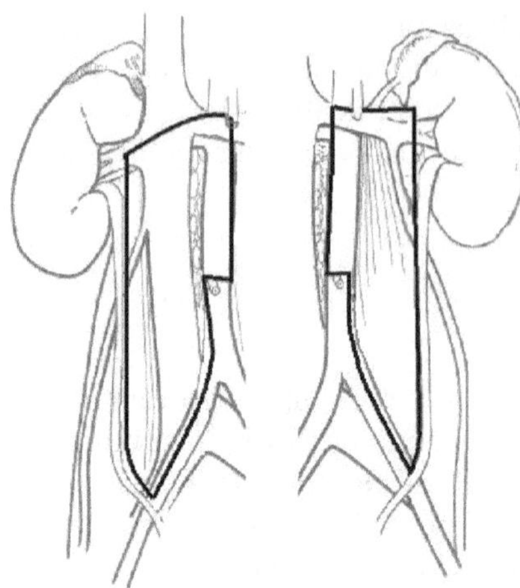

Fig. 1. Retroperitoneal template for laparoscopic lymph node dissection

toneum whereas a Hasson cannula is used if indicated. The first trocar is placed at the umbilicus for the laparoscope whereas two secondary trocars are placed at the lateral edge of the rectus muscle 8 cm above and below the umbilicus for the surgeons' instruments. A fourth trocar is placed at the anterior axillary line in the best point for retraction decided by the surgeon. Five- and 10-mm trocars are used.

Right Side

The peritoneum is incised at the internal inguinal ring then along the line of Toldt from the cecum to the right colic flexure. Cephalic dissection is carried out parallel to the transverse colon and lateral to the duodenum along the vena cava up to the hepatoduodenal ligament, while the caudal dissection is continued along the spermatic vessels down to the internal inguinal ring. In the next step the colon, duodenum, and the head of pancreas are reflected medially until the anterior surface of the vena cava, aorta, and left renal vein are completely exposed (Fig. 2). The spermatic vein is dissected free along its entire course and excised. Then the spermatic artery is clipped and transected at its crossing over the vena cava whereas spermatic artery origin will be approached later.

Cranial to caudal the lymphatic tissue overlying the vena cava is split open, then the lateral and anterior surfaces of the vena cava are dissected free. Both renal veins are then dissected free (Fig. 3). Lymphatic tissue overlying the right common iliac artery is incised and the dissection is continued from caudal in a cephalic direction up to the origin of the inferior mesenteric artery. Cephalic to the inferior mesenteric artery dissection is continued upward along the left margin to the aorta, thereby the ventral surface of the aorta is completely freed. Then the spermatic artery is clipped at its origin.

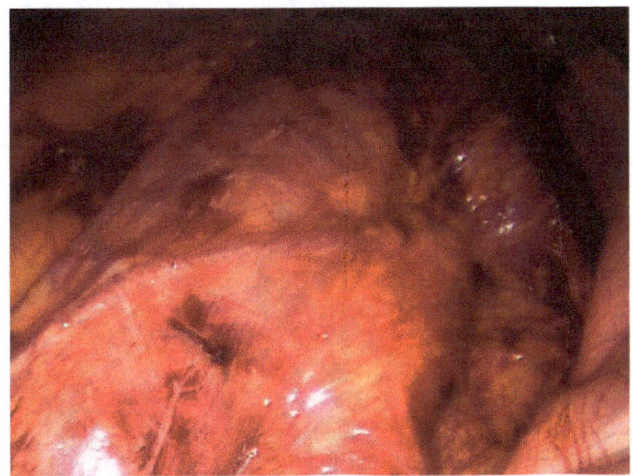

FIG. 2. Wide exposure of the right retroperitoneum. From *right to left*: the duodenum is reflected; left renal vein, aorta and vena cava covered with posterior peritoneum. In the *middle* of the picture the gonadal artery crosses the vena cava anteriorly

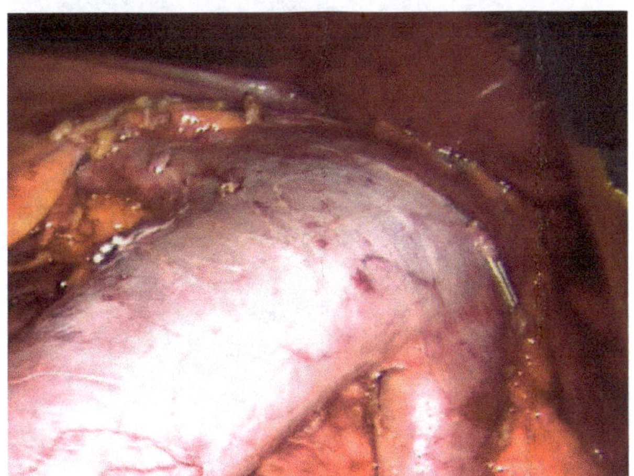

FIG. 3. Posterior peritoneum is dissected until the vena cava and both renal veins are dissected free

Cranial to caudal the interaortocaval space is then dissected, starting from the lower edge of the right renal artery down to the lumbar vessels, and the lymphatic tissue is removed step by step (Fig. 4). The right renal vein and artery lateral to the vena cava delineate the cranial border of the dissection, while the caudal border of the dissection is the point where the ureter crosses the iliac vessels (Figs. 5 and 6). The lymphatic tissue is clipped distally then the dissection is continued cephalic until the lymphatic package is freed, while the lumbar veins are exposed, but they are only transected in exceptional cases. Lymph nodes lateral to the vena cava and medial to the ureter are dissected free, then the nodal package can be removed within a specimen retrieval bag. The colon and duodenum are returned to their anatomic position and secured with one suture

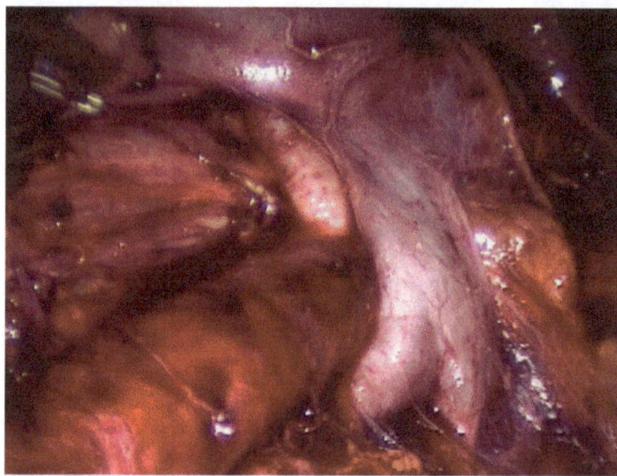

FIG. 4. The space is completely free of lymphatic tissue. The left renal vein and the right renal artery are the upper limit of dissection. The spine is seen in the interaortocaval space

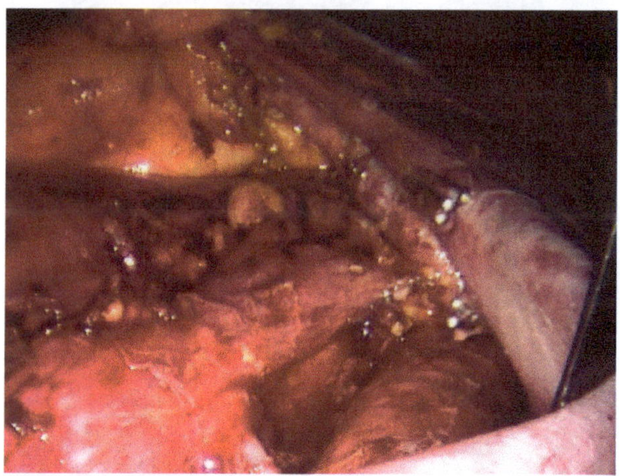

FIG. 5. The vena cava is retracted medially and the aorta is seen underneath. The right renal vein and artery define the upper limit of dissection. The entire interaortocaval and the tissue lateral to the vena cava are removed. A clipped lumbar vein is seen on the lateral side of vena cava

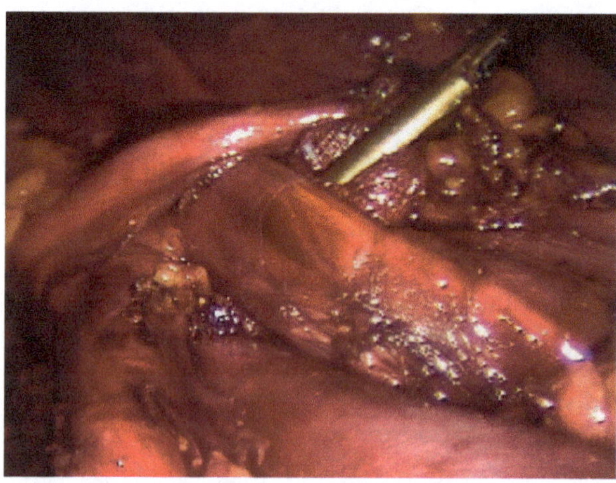

FIG. 6. Lower limit of dissection for the right template. The ureter is seen in the *upper left corner* of the picture crossing the common iliac vessels

laterally, which is tied extracorporeally. Drains are not used to avoid lymphocele formation.

Left Side

The peritoneum is incised along the line of Toldt starting from the left colonic flexure down to the pelvic brim and distally along the spermatic vein to the internal inguinal ring. The splenocolic ligament is transected and the colon is dissected until the anterior surface of the aorta is exposed. In the next step the spermatic vein is dissected along its entire course and excised, then the ureter is identified laterally and separated from the lymphatic tissue carefully to preserve its blood supply. That step will facilitate left renal vein dissection until it is freed completely (Fig. 7).

Dissection of the lymphatic template is started caudally at the crossing of the ureter with the common iliac vessels by splitting the lymphatic tissue over the anterior surface of the left common iliac artery in a cephalic direction along the lateral border of the aorta, circumventing the inferior mesenteric artery on the left side and preserving it. Cephalic to the inferior mesenteric artery dissection is continued along the anterior and medial surfaces of the aorta up to the left renal vein, and during this dissection the origin of the spermatic artery is clipped and transected. Next to that the lateral surface of the aorta is dissected down to the origin of the lumbar arteries. To gain access to the left renal artery the lumbar vein draining into the left renal vein must be transected (Fig. 8). Other lumbar vessels are dissected free from the lymphatic tissue to the point at which they disappear in the layer between the spine and psoas muscle (Fig. 9), then the sympathetic chain lateral to that point can be identified.

When the nodal package is completely freed, it can be retrieved within a laparoscopic retrieval bag. Then the colon is secured in its anatomic position with an extracorporeally tied suture. Drains are not used.

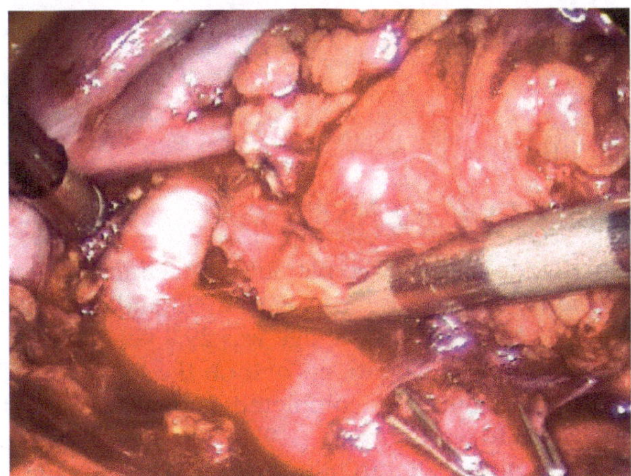

FIG. 7. Left template dissection: the anterior wall of the aorta is exposed with clipped gonadal artery. In the *upper left corner* of the picture the renal artery and vein delineate the upper limit of dissection. Lymphatic package is seen lateral to the aorta

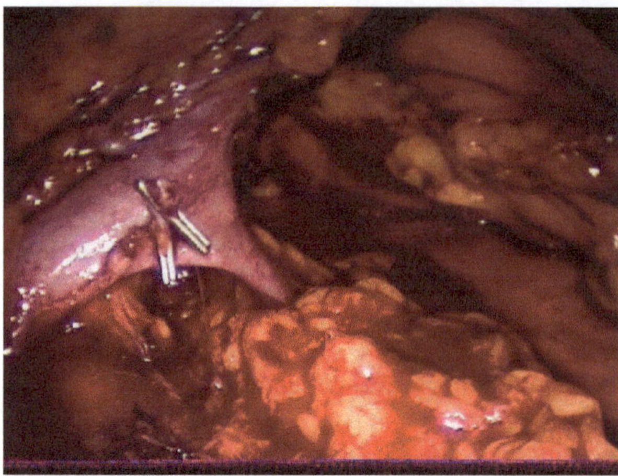

FIG. 8. Lumbar vein draining into left renal vein and a clipped gonadal vein

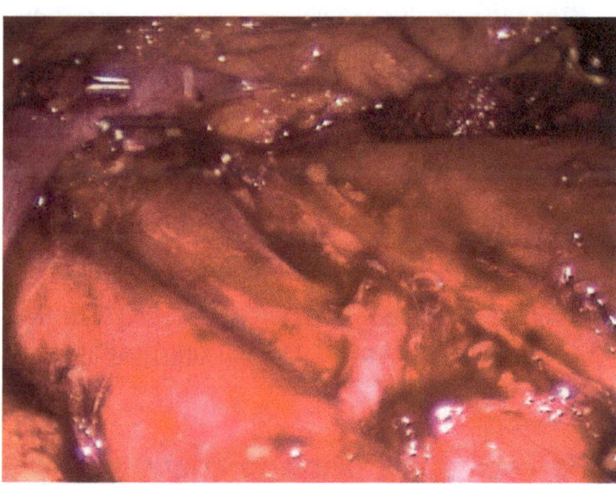

FIG. 9. Surgical template after left laparoscopic retrosperitoneal lymph node dissection. *Left upper corner*: left renal vein; *right lower corner*: aorta. *Middle of picture*: a lumbar artery disappears between the spine and the psoas muscle

Results

Clinical Stage I NSGCT

One hundred and three patients with clinical stage I disease underwent laparoscopic RPLND between August 1992 and June 2004 with a mean follow-up of 62 (6–113) months. Mean age was 29.9 years (16–51). The tumor was located on the right side in 64 patients and on the left side in 39 patients.

The procedure was completed as planned in all but three patients who were converted to open surgery (2.9%). Conversion was due to injury of a small aortic branch, another due to injury of renal vein in a horseshoe kidney, and the third due to injury of a left renal vein ventral to the aorta. Four other minor intraoperative complications were encountered including vena cava, renal vein, and lumbar vein injuries. All were controlled laparoscopically with either clips or fibrin glue; a left renal vein injury was controlled via laparoscopic suturing. Few minor complications occurred postoperatively including three asymptomatic lymphoceles, a transient irritation of the genitofemoral nerve, and a spontaneously resolving retroperitoneal hematoma.

Once the learning curve was overcome the average operative time was 217 min on exclusion of the first 30 patients. Mean blood loss was 144 ml (range 10–500), not including 2600 ml in a converted patient with a horseshoe kidney. Mean postoperative hospitalization was 3.6 (range 2–8) days.

Twenty-six of 103 patients had an active tumor in the resected retroperitoneal lymph nodes, and were therefore treated with adjuvant chemotherapy. During their follow-up there was not a single recurrence observed. Seventy-seven of 103 patients had no tumor in the resected retroperitoneal lymph nodes, and five relapses were observed. One retroperitoneal recurrence occurred on the contralateral side outside the surgical field. Further investigations revealed that the tumor in the resected retroperitoneal lymph nodes was missed on histological examination. This patient was cured with two cycles of chemotherapy and contralateral laparoscopic RPLND. Three other patients developed lung recurrences. Another patient had elevation of his tumor markers without identifiable recurrence site.

A sixth patient who was treated in another center by primary chemotherapy developed retroperitoneal relapse after1 year of follow-up with negative tumor markers. Laparoscopic RPLND was performed and the pathology revealed mature teratoma with immature ectodermal elements. Therefore, this patient was treated with two cycles of adjuvant chemotherapy and he is free of recurrence during 16 months of follow-up. No further relapses occurred.

In 100 of our patients, antegrade ejaculation was preserved while three patients missed their follow-up.

Clinical Stage II NSGCT

Between February 1995 and June 2004, 59 patients with clinical stage II disease underwent laparoscopic RPLND after primary chemotherapy (43 stage IIB and 16 stage IIC). The mean age was 29.2 (15–56) years. The procedure was performed on the right side in 32 patients and on the left side in 27. The mean follow-up was 53 (10–89) months.

No conversion occurred and the spectrum of complications was almost the same as stage I patients, with a higher incidence of chylous ascites in stage II. The mean operative time was 234 (135–360) min and the mean blood loss was 165 (20–350) ml. Postoperative hospital stay averaged 3.8 (3–10) days.

Of the 43 patients with clinical stage IIB, 16 had mature teratomas and 26 had no tumor in the resected lymph nodes. One patient had an active tumor which was a borderline case between stage IIB and IIC. One patient with stage IIB disease had recurrence after 24 months of follow-up which was outside the surgical field at the external iliac lymph nodes close to the internal inguinal ring. This recurrence was again resected laparoscopically. The pathology of this node was mature teratoma, which was followed, and no further relapse was observed with a follow-up of 8 months.

Of the 16 patients with clinical stage IIC, 10 had no tumor and 5 had mature teratomas. One patient had seminoma clinical stage IIC, which was treated by three cycles of chemotherapy. The size of the retroperitoneal tumor mass decreased to 20% of its original size (from 30cm down to 6cm). Clinically, there was no change in the size of the retroperitoneal mass after the second cycle of chemotherapy. A positron emission tomography scan was done and was negative. Laparoscopic RPLND was then performed and the pathology of the resected mass showed foci of viable tumor. The patient was treated with two more cycles of chemotherapy and is free of relapse with a follow-up of 3 years.

In 57 of our patients, antegrade ejaculation was preserved while two patients lost their antegrade ejaculation.

Discussion

Retroperitoneal lymph node dissection in the management of nonseminomatous germ cell tumors of the testis has been always favored in our practice because it has a high diagnostic accuracy and its immediate stratification for further treatment options, i.e., adjuvant chemotherapy or surveillance. Relapse rates after open RPLND alone are as high as 8%–29% for stage I Ia tumors [7,8] and 34%–55% for stage I Ib tumors [8,9]. This rate falls to as low as 0%–1% if two cycles of adjuvant chemotherapy are given [9,10], therefore all of our clinical stage I patients diagnosed as pathological stage II following open RPLND received chemotherapy as the definitive treatment.

Looking at our results for stage I disease alongside similar studies conducted by Steiner et al. [1], Castillo et al. [11], Rassweiler et al. [3], and Bhayani et al. [12] (Tables 1 and 2), they were comparable in all intraoperative and postoperative parameters and in comparison to the open surgical RPLND, laparoscopy technically duplicated the open surgical technique in a comparable operative time but showed less postoperative morbidity, quicker convalescence, and improved cosmetic results [1–4,13]. In all of those series oncologic efficiency of the procedure was proven.

The oncologic efficiency of our procedure was compared with that of the open technique. Of 239 NSGCT clinical stage I patients, 172 were identified as pathological stage I in a recent series of open RPLND [14]. A retroperitoneal relapse rate of 1.2% was observed in this group, while our relapse rate of 1.15% compares favorably with that of open surgery and clearly demonstrates its oncologic efficacy.

Our results for stage II disease were again compared to similar studies conducted by Steiner et al. [1], Castillo et al. [12], Rassweiler et al. [15], and Palese

Table 1. Clinical stage I operative data

First author [Ref.]	No. of cases	Approach	Operative time (min)	Blood loss (ml)	No. of conversions	Intraoperative complications		Postoperative complications		Hospital stay (days)
						Major	Minor	Major	Minor	
Janetschek [this study]	103	Transperitoneal	217	144	3	3	4	0	5	3.6
Castillo [11]	96[a]	Transperitoneal	138	120	4	4	5	1	4	1.8
Rassweiler [3]	34[b]	17 → Transperitoneal	248	—	1	1	—	2	5	5.3
Bhayani [12]	29	Transperitoneal	258	241	2	—	—	—	2	2.6

[a] All intraoperative data and postoperative complications were calculated on 128 patients (96 clinical stage I + 20 IIA + 12 IIB). The approach was extraperitoneal in 5 patients.
[b] The procedure was abandoned in 3 patients, 4 had seminoma, 2 had Leydig cell carcinoma, and 17 patients underwent extraperitoneal approach.

Table 2. Clinical stage I follow-up

First author [Ref.]	No. of cases		Clinical stage	Pathological stage	Adjuvant chemotherapy	Follow-up (months)	No. of relapses	
							Retroperitoneal	Other
Janetschek [this study]	103	77	I	I	No	62	1 → contralateral side	4
		26	I	II	2 × BEP	62	0	0
Castillo [11]	96	78	I	I	—	34	4 → site of relapse not clear	
		18	I	II	—			
Rassweiler [3]	34[a]	28	I	I	No	40	0	2
		6	I	II	3 × BEP	40	0	0
Bhayani [12]	29	17	I	I	No	69.6	0	2
		12[b]	I	II	2 × BEP	75.6	0	1[b]

[a] Results were for the transperitoneal and the extraperitoneal approach.
[b] Two patients refused chemotherapy, but only one of them relapsed.

et al. [16] (Tables 3 and 4). It is very obvious that this is a technically demanding procedure and carries substantial complications, but it was proven to be feasible. Oncologic efficiency of the procedure is clearly seen in all series.

In our series there was one patient with seminoma stage IIC who underwent laparoscopic RPLND. There is a general consensus that there is no place for RPLND in the management of seminoma clinical stage I since the morbidities of alternative therapies are low and their efficacy is very high [17]. On the other hand, RPLND is considered to remove residual retroperitoneal masses after chemotherapy in exceptional cases of seminoma, which was proven to be feasible by laparoscopic means.

Loss of antegrade ejaculation is the major long-term morbidity encountered after RPLND. This drawback can be overcome either by performing a template dissection as described by Weissbach and Boedefeld [6] or by nerve-sparing RPLND [18]. In clinical stage I the template dissection downscales the operative field yet maintains acceptable sensitivity and, more importantly, does not increase relapse. We have followed this strategy in our work and in 100 of our stage I patients, antegrade ejaculation was preserved while three patients were lost during follow-up. In stage II patients, antegrade ejaculation was preserved in 57 of 59 patients.

With the introduction of nerve-sparing RPLND, Donohue's group was able to improve the ejaculation rate from 70% to almost 100%. However, Donohue did not only introduce nerve-sparing dissection but also simultaneously limited the dissection to the unilateral template described by Weissbach et al. [8,18].Using this template the contralateral sympathetic nerves remain intact and it has been known since 1951 that destruction of the sympathetic chain on one side does not result in aspermia [19]. Therefore, nerve sparing in addition to a unilateral template dissection is not necessary at all as it cannot improve on the good results for antegrade ejaculation preservation which is already achieved by unilateral template dissection alone. Obviously, template dissection can be performed more precisely with laparoscopy than with open surgery, since the anatomy is not disturbed by retractors.

Peschel et al. have shown that nerve-sparing RPLND is feasible by means of laparoscopy. They published an average operative time of 3.2h, a blood loss of 66ml, and a hospital stay of 3.7 days in five patients [20]. This required meticulous dissection and identification of the sympathetic chain and the postganglionic fibers in the retrocaval, interaortocaval, and para-aortic regions. Although, as we mentioned, antegrade ejaculation is routinely preserved when a nerve-sparing dissection is limited to a unilateral template, the development of a unilateral laparoscopic nerve-sparing technique is a step toward bilateral laparoscopic dissection.

The overall costs of laparoscopic RPLND including surgery and hospitalization were slightly lower than those of open RPLND during our evaluation [21], while they were slightly higher in another study [22]. This is due to many possible reasons such as cost and length of hospitalization, operative time cost,

TABLE 3. Clinical stage II operative data

First author [Ref.]	No. of cases	Clinical stage	Primary chemo.	Approach	Operative time (min)	Blood loss (ml)	No. of conversions	Intraoperative complications		Postoperative complications		Hospital stay (days)
								Major	Minor	Major	Minor	
Janetschek [this study]	59	43 IIB 16 IIC[a]	2 × BEP 3 × BEP	Transperitoneal	216 281	165	0	0	9[a]	0	11[a]	3.8
Steiner [1]	72	4 IIA 10 IIA 43 IIB 15 IIC	No 2 × BEP 2 × BEP 3 × BEP	Transperitoneal	243	78	0	2[b]	—	—	25[b]	3.7
Castillo [11]	32	20 IIA 12 IIB	—	Transperitoneal[c]	138	120	4	4	5	1	4	1.8
Rassweiler [15]	8[d]	2 IIB 6 IIC	? × BEP ? × BEP	Transperitoneal	348 362	—	0 6	—	—	—	1	3.5 8.2
Palese [16]	7[e]	≥IIA	3–4 × BEP	Transperitoneal	318	344	2	3	1	3	—	2

[a] One patient had seminoma stage IIC, 9 Intraoperative bleedings managed laparoscopically and 11 minor postoperative complications (7 chylous ascites + 4 asymptomatic lymphoceles).

[b] Two major intraoperative complications (colon + renal artery injuries). 25 minor postoperative complications (9 chylous ascites + 16 asymptomatic lymphoceles) are calculated on 185 patients (113 stage I + 72 stages II).

[c] All intraoperative data and postoperative complications were calculated on 128 patients (96 clinical stage I + 20 IIA + 12 IIB). The approach was extraperitoneal in 5 patients.

[d] All patients had post chemotherapy residual retroperitoneal mass.

[e] All patients had postchemotherapy residual retroperitoneal mass or prechemotherapy mass size >3.0 cm. One patient had seminoma and 1 had epididymal small cell tumor. Intraoperative complications were vascular.

TABLE 4. Clinical stage II follow-up

First author [Ref.]	No. of cases	Clinical stage	Primary chemo.	Vital tumors	Follow-up (months)	No. of relapses	
						Retroperitoneal	Others
Janetschek [this study]	59	43 IIB	2 × BEP	1[a,c]	53	1 → stage IIB (external iliac LN)	0
		16 IIC	3 × BEP	1[b]			
Steiner [1]	72	4 IIA	No	2[c]	57.6	0	0
		10 IIA	2 × BEP	0		0	0
		43 IIB	2 × BEP	0		0	0
		15 IIC	3 × BEP	1[c]		1 → retrocaval	0
Castillo [11]	32	20 IIA	—	—	34	2 → site of relapse not clear	
		12 IIB				3 → site of relapse not clear	
Rassweiler [15]	8	2 IIB	? × BEP	0	29	0	0
		6 IIC	? × BEP	0		0	0
Palese [16]	7	≥IIA	3–4 × BEP	2[c]	24	0	0

[a] A borderline case between stage IIB and IIC.
[b] One case of seminoma.
[c] Patients with vital tumor in the specimen received adjuvant chemotherapy.

amount of disposables used during laparoscopy, and the comparison of relatively new evolving technology with well-established procedure. Patient satisfaction, however, was clearly higher with laparoscopic RPLND than with open RPLND, which was demonstrated in an extensive quality-of-life study [23].

In conclusion, laparoscopic RPLND has demonstrated its surgical and oncologic efficacy. The morbidity and the complication rate are low. Adherence to the templates previously described allows for preservation of antegrade ejaculation in virtually all patients. It is indeed a difficult procedure, but once the long and steep learning curve has been overcome, operative times are equal to or even shorter than those of open surgery. Thereafter, the costs will be within the range of those for open surgery. Survival and tumor recurrence rate after laparoscopic RPLND are at least as low and equal to that of open surgery. Patient satisfaction, however, is clearly higher with laparoscopic RPLND.

References

1. Steiner H, Peschel R, Janetschek G, Holtl L, Berger AP, Bartsch G, Hobisch A (2004) Long-term result of laparoscopic retroperitoneal lymph node dissection: a single-center 10 years experience. Urology 63:550–555
2. Corvin S, Kuczyk M, Anastasiadis A, Stenzl A (2004) Laparoscopic retroperitoneal lymph node dissection for nonseminomatous testicular carcinoma. World J Urol 22:33–36

3. Rassweiler JJ, Frede T, Lenz E, Seemann O, Alken P (2000) Long-term experience with laparoscopic retroperitoneal lymph node dissection in the management of low-stage testis cancer. Eur Urol 37:251–260
4. Bhayani SB, Allaf ME, Kavoussi LR (2004) Laparoscopic retroperitoneal lymph node dissection for clinical stage I nonseminomatous germ cell testicular cancer: current status. Urol Oncol 22:145–148
5. Klingler HC, Remzi M, Janetschek G, Marberger M (2003) Benefits of laparoscopic renal surgery are more pronounced in patients with a high body mass index. Eur Urol 43:522–527
6. Weissbach L, Boedefeld EA (1987) Testicular tumour study group: localization of solitary and multiple metastases in stage II non seminomatous testis tumour as basis for modified staging lymph node dissection in stage I. J Urol 138:77–82
7. Richie JP, Kantoff PW (1991) Is adjuvant chemotherapy necessary for patients with stage BI testicular cancer? J Clin Oncol 9:1393–1396
8. Donhue JP, Thornhill JA, Foster RS, Roland RG, Bihrle R (1993) Retroperitoneal lymphadenectomy for clinical stage A testis cancer (1965–1989): modification of technique and impact on ejaculation. J Urol 149:243–237
9. Williams SD, Stablein DM, Einhorn LH, Muggia FM, Weiss RB, Donohue JP, Paulson DF, Brunner KW, Jacobs EM, Spaulding JT (1987) Immediate adjuvant chemotherapy versus observation with treatment at relapse in pathological stage II testicular cancer. N Engl J Med 317:1433–1438
10. Javadpour N (1984) Predictors of recurrence in stage II nonseminomatous testicular cancer after lymphadenectomy: implications for adjuvant chemotherapy. J Urol 135:629
11. Castillo O, Urena R, Pinto I, Olivares R, Portalier P (2004) Laparoscopic retroperitoneal lymph node dissection for stage I and II NSGCT. J Urol Suppl number 933, Volum 171, page 247–248.
12. Bhayani SB, Ong A, Oh WK, Kantoff PW, Kavoussi LR (2003) Laparoscopic retroperitoneal lymph node dissection for clinical stage I nonseminomatous germ cell testicular cancer: A long-term update. Urology 62:324–327
13. Janetschek G, Hobisch A, Höltl L, Bartsch G (1996) Retroperitoneal lymphadenectomy for clinical stage I nonseminomatous testicular tumor: Laparoscopy versus open surgery and impact of learning curve. J Urol 156:89–93
14. Heidenreich A, Albers P, Hartmann M, Kliesch S, Koehrmann K, Krege S, Lossin P, Weissbach L (2003) Complications of nerve sparing retroperitoneal lymph node dissection for clinical stage I nonseminomatous germ cell tumours of the testis (Experience of the German testicular cancer study group). J Urol 169:1710–1714
15. Rassweiler JJ, Seemann O, Henkel TO, Stock C, Frede T, Alken P (1996) Laparoscopic retroperitoneal lymph node dissection for non seminomatous germ cell tumour: indication and limitation. J Urol 156:1108–1113
16. Palese MA, Li-Ming Su, Kavoussi LR (2002) laparoscopic retroperitoneal lymph node dissection after chemotherapy. Urology 60:130–134
17. Steiner H, Holtl L, Wirtenberger W, Berger AP, Bartsch G, Hobisch A (2002) Long-term experience with carboplatin monotherapy for clinical stage I seminoma: a retrospective single-center study. Urology 60:324–328
18. Donohue JP, Foster RS, Rowland RG, Bihrle R, Jones J, Geier G (1990) Nerve-sparing retroperitoneal lymphadenectomy with preservation of ejaculation. J Urol 144:287–291

19. Whitelaw GP, Smithwick RH (1951) Some secondary effects of sympathectomy with particular reference to disturbance of sexual function. N Engl J Med 245:212
20. Peschel R, Gettman MT, Neururer R, Hobisch A, Bartsch G (2002) Laparoscopic retroperitoneal lymph node dissection: Description of the nerve sparing technique. Urology 60:339–343
21. Janetschek G (2001) Laparoscopic RPLND. Urol Clin North Am 28:107–114
22. Ogan K, Lotan Y, Koeneman K, Pearle MS, Cadeddu JA, Rassweiler J (2002) Laparoscopic versus open retroperitoneal lymph node dissection: a cost analysis. J Urol 168:1945–1949
23. Hobisch A, Tönnemann J, Janetschek G (1998) Morbidity and quality of life after open versus laparoscopic retroperitoneal lymphadenectomy for testicular tumour—the patient's view. In: Jones WG, Appleyard I, Harnden P, Joffe JK (eds) Germ cell tumours VI. John Libbey, London, p 277

Laparoscopic Retroperitoneal Lymph Node Dissection: Extraperitoneal Approach

Makoto Satoh, Akihiro Ito, and Yoichi Arai

Summary. We review our early experience with laparoscopic retroperitoneal lymph node dissection (RPLND) via extraperitoneal approach to assess the precise pathological status of retroperitoneal lymph nodes in early-stage testicular cancer. A total of 32 patients (23 with stage I, 4 with stage IIa, and 5 with stage IIb) with testicular cancer underwent extraperitoneal laparoscopic RPLND in the supine position. After developing the sufficient retroperitoneal space, the modified unilateral retroperitoneal lymph node dissection was performed. For stage I cases, a gamma probe guided laparoscopic RPLND was performed. The mean operating time for laparoscopy was 209 min (median 222, range 131–372 min). Mean blood loss was 44 ml (median 10, range scarce to 260 ml). There was no open conversion. Two patients had prolonged lymph drainage (more than 7 days). One had a symptomatic lymphocyst treated with laparoscopic fenestration. In one case, a segmental renal infarction was noted after the operation. In 13 recent cases, the ipsilateral lumbar sympathetic nerves relevant to ejaculation were preserved and functional preservation was confirmed by intraoperative electrostimulation. Micrometastasis was found in three of clinical stage I and one of stage IIA disease. Extraperitoneal laparoscopic RPLND is technically feasible and decreases postoperative morbidity.

Keywords. Testicular cancer, Retroperitoneal lymph node dissection, Extraperitoneal laparoscopy, Sentinel lymph node, Gamma probe

Introduction

The optimal post-orchiectomy management of early-stage nonseminomatous testicular tumor is a controversial issue in urology. Some authors advocate ongoing surveillance because of the efficacy of chemotherapy in testicular

Department of Urology, Tohoku University School of Medicine, 1-1 Seiryo-machi, Aoba-ku, Sendai 980-8574, Japan

cancer, but such a strategy also requires optimal patient compliance [1]. Other authors [2,3] prefer a modified, nerve-sparing lymphadenectomy on the grounds of early detection and subsequent chemotherapy of retroperitoneal micrometastases, which may already exist in approximately 30% of these patients [4].

For stage I seminoma, the management is also controversial. Because there are no effective tumor markers for seminoma, the early detection of metastasis is difficult in surveillance follow-up. The recurrence rates of stage I seminoma have ranged from 9% to 23% [6]. Some authors advocate adjuvant radiotherapy for stage I seminoma [7], but such treatment for retroperitoneal lymph nodes may lead to gastrointestinal symptoms, peptic ulceration, aspermia, and the possible induction of secondary malignancies on long-term follow-up [8–10].

In stage II disease, retroperitoneal lymph node dissection (RPLND) can be performed as a first line of treatment or after chemotherapy; the latter approach confers a staging benefit because patients with active tumor receive adjuvant chemotherapy postoperatively. On the other hand, the morbidity of open retroperitoneal lymphadenectomy for stage I testicular tumor is too high for the staging technique. If an easy and safe laparoscopic RPLND method were developed, it might offer the possibility of exact lymph node staging to avoid overtreatment of true stage I testicular tumor.

Recently, laparoscopic RPLND has been gaining popularity as a minimally invasive staging surgery [11–13]. We present the simplified surgical technique via the extraperitoneal approach in the supine position, as well as the morbidity and convalescence of this procedure.

Patients and Methods

Patients

From January 2002 to November 2004, a total of 32 patients (23 with stage I, 4 with stage IIa, and 5 with stage IIb) with testicular cancer underwent extraperitoneal laparoscopic RPLND in the supine position. For three of 4 stage IIa and all of stage IIb patients, laparoscopic RPLND was performed after cisplatin-based chemotherapy. The median age of the patients was 34 (range 21–53) years (Table 1).

Operative Technique

The surgical procedure consisted of two phases. The first phase involved development of sufficient retroperitoneal space with blunt dissection and carbon dioxide instillation. After widely extending the retroperitoneal space, the surgeon can see a dome, having a ceiling of peritoneum with the ureter and testicular vein and the floor of the great vessels. The second phase was a procedure based on a unilateral template lymphadenectomy, the technique of which is almost same as open conventional surgery [14]. On the right side, the template

TABLE 1. Characteristics of the 32 patients

Median age, years (range)	34 (21–53)
Side of testicular cancer	
Left	18
Right	14
Pathology of testicular cancer	
Seminoma	20
Nonseminoma	12
Clinical stage	
I	23
IIa	4
IIb	5

included the tissue ventral to the vena cava, the right paracaval, and the interaortocaval tissue. The cranial border of the dissection was the renal vessels, and the caudal border was the bifurcation of the common iliac artery. The template for the right side was substantially similar to that for the left side. It included the all tissue lateral and ventral to the aorta, and interaortocaval tissue between the renal vessels and the origin of the inferior mesenteric artery. In our laparoscopic procedure, great attention should be given to making a large retroperitoneal space without injuring the peritoneum.

Position and Port Placement

Under general anesthesia, the patient was placed in the supine position and was moved to the operator side edge of the operating table. The surgeon stood on the same side as the tumor, cephalad to an assistant who held the camera. A small incision was made at a third lateral point on the line between the navel and iliac crest. After blunt splitting of muscles, the index finger was inserted into the preperitoneal space, and the peritoneum was separated from abdominal muscles. A PDB balloon dissecting trocar (US Surgical, Norwalk, CT, USA) with an endoscope was inserted, and the extraperitoneal space was extended with instillation of 500ml of air under endoscopic monitoring. After removing the balloon dissecting trocar, the endoscope was introduced via this port, and carbon dioxide was instilled into the space. Two other lateral trocars were inserted on the anterior axillary line under endoscopic view with great attention being paid to avoiding injury to the peritoneum. If necessary, an additional fourth trocar was inserted caudal to the first port under endoscopic view (Figs. 1 and 2).

Extension of Retroperitoneal Space

After the establishment of a pneumoretroperitoneal space with a maximum CO_2 pressure of 8mmHg, the laterocoronal fascia was dissected upward on the psoas muscle and fatty tissues on this muscle were lifted up with blunt dissection. The

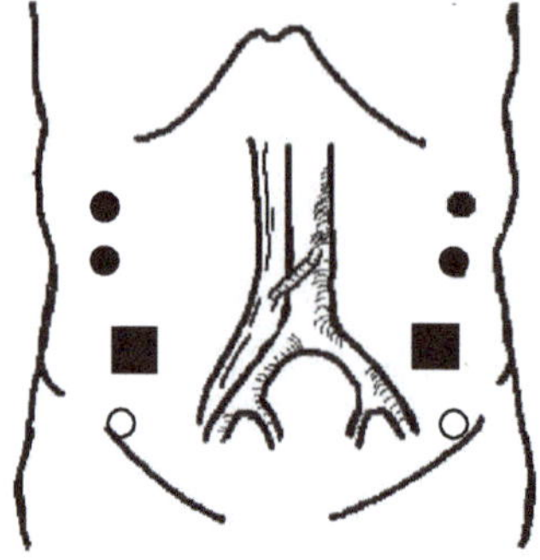

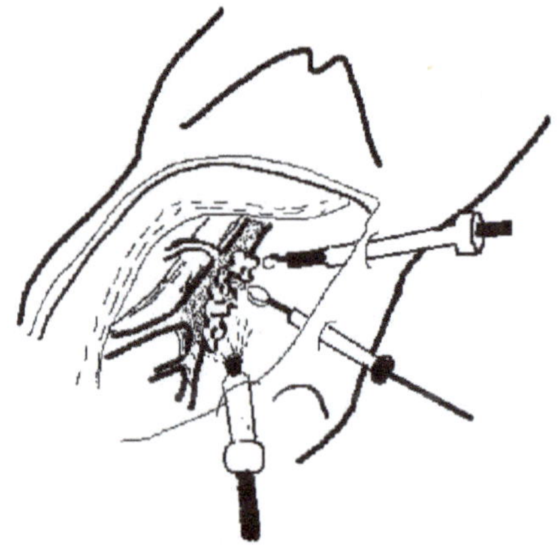

Fig. 1. The site of trocar placement and schema of extending the retroperitoneal space. *Squares*, 12 mm trocar for camera; *closed circles*, 12 mm or 5 mm trocar. If necessary, an additional trocar (*open circle*) was inserted caudal to the first port under endoscopic view. With the blunt dissection of adequate plane and insufflation of carbon dioxide, the retroperitoneal space was widely and easily extended

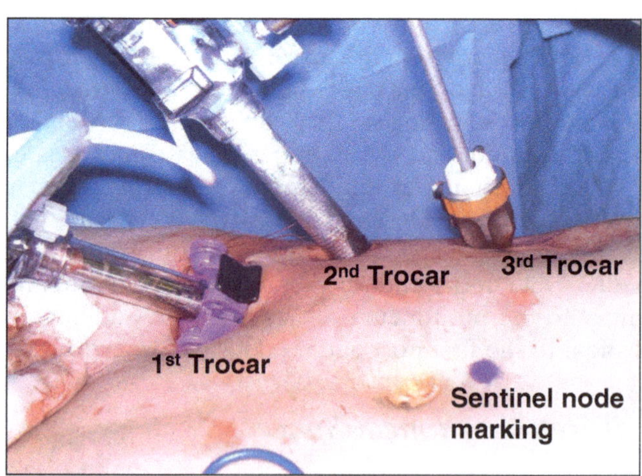

Fig. 2. The site of trocar placement, and preoperative sentinel lymph node marking (left side tumor)

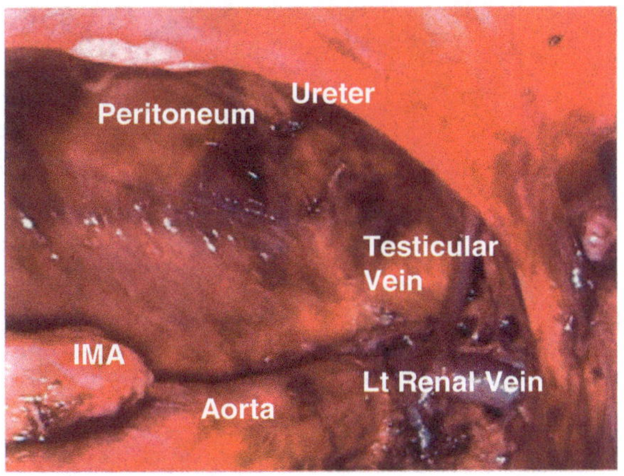

Fig. 3. The retroperitoneal space was extended widely like a dome, having a peritoneal ceiling with the ureter and the spermatic vein adding to the effect of carbon dioxide insufflation and allowing retraction of the peritoneum. *IMA*, inferior mesenteric artery

ureter and the spermatic vein were identified on the surface of the common iliac artery or psoas muscle and then were lifted up together with the peritoneum and retracted anteromedially.

The space between the peritoneum and the common iliac artery was separated with a blunt dissection. In the left case, this dissection was continued to the left lateral surface of the aorta, the anterior surface of the aorta, and the vena cava above the origin of the inferior mesenteric artery, to the left renal vein. In the right case, this dissection was continued to the lateral and anterior surface of the vena cava, the right lateral surface of the aorta, the anterior surface of the aorta above the origin of the inferior mesenteric artery, and the left renal vein.

Thus the retroperitoneal space was extended widely like a dome, having a peritoneal ceiling with the ureter and the spermatic vein, and a floor containing the anterior surface of the aorta, the inferior mesenteric artery, the common iliac artery, and the vena cava, adding to the effect of carbon dioxide insufflation allowing retraction of the peritoneum (Fig. 3).

Lymph Node Dissection with Modified Unilateral Template

The retroperitoneal lymph node within the modified unilateral template was removed [14]. For stage I testicular cancer cases, one day before surgery, 15 MBq of technetium-99m-labeled phylate in 0.4 ml of saline was injected around the tumor inside the testicular tunica albuginea with a 29-gauge butterfly needle. Detailed lymph node mapping procedures were reported previously [15]. In these cases, after the radical orchiectomy, gamma probe-guided extraperitoneal laparoscopic RPLND was performed. The location of sentinel lymph nodes was confirmed by gamma probe navigation [16] (Fig. 4).

The lymphadenectomy was started from the bifurcation of the common iliac artery on the ipsilateral side, extended cephalad. To prevent postoperative lymphorrhea, the efferent lymph vessels were controlled by hemostatic clips [17].

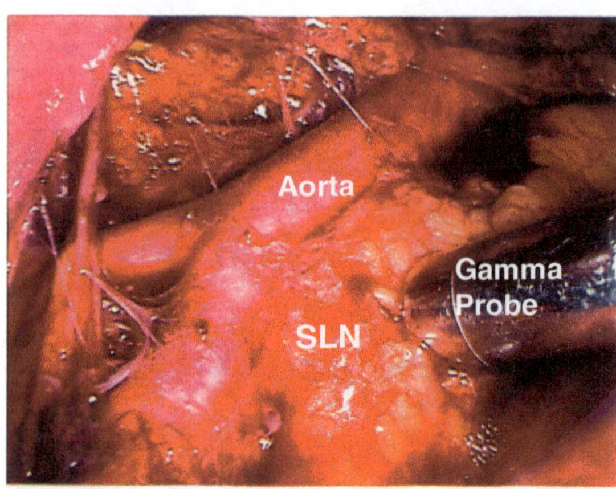

FIG. 4. The location of sentinel lymph nodes was confirmed by gamma probe. *SLN*, sentinel lymph node

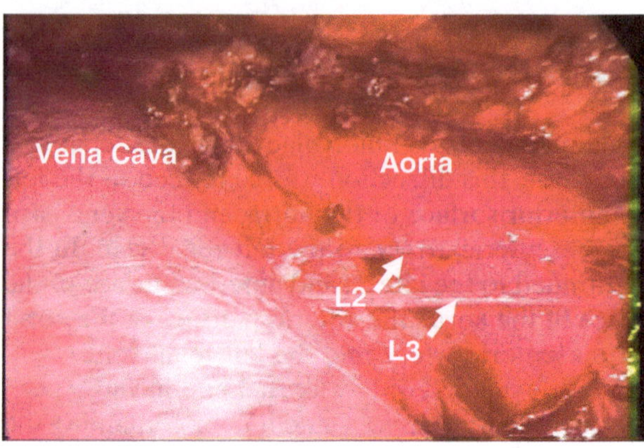

FIG. 5. The ipsilateral postganglionic nerves arising from the L2 or L3 (*arrows*) sympathetic ganglia were preserved (right side tumor)

The interaortocaval nodes were removed. Since the primary landing sites were reported to be invariably located ventrally, the retrocaval and retroaortic nodes were not removed in our procedure [18]. The ipsilateral spermatic veins were removed in their entirety. In this template lymph node dissection, the contralateral ejaculatory nerves were preserved. In a recent series of 12 stage I patients, the ipsilateral postganglionic nerves arising from the L2 or L3 sympathetic ganglia were preserved [19] (Fig. 5).

Results

A total of 32 patients underwent this operative procedure. Mean operating time for lymphadenectomy was 209 min (range 131–372 min). Mean blood loss was 44 ml (median 10, range scarce to 260 ml). There was no open conversion.

There was peritoneal penetration during developing retroperitoneal space in four of the first 14 cases and two of the most recent 16 cases. Postoperative symptomatic lymphocyst was observed in one case and was treated with laparoscopic fenestration. Prolonged lymphorrhea was observed in three cases. In one case of clinical stage IIa, an accessory polar artery was injured intraoperatively and a small segmental renal infarction was recognized by computed tomography scan after the operation. All patients started to walk and have oral intake on the day following the operation (Table 2).

Micrometastasis of lymph node was found in four cases (three of clinical stage I and one of stage IIa disease) and conventional chemotherapy was performed for four such patients. In 12 recent cases, the ipsilateral lumbar sympathetic nerves relevant to ejaculation were preserved and functional preservation was confirmed by intraoperative electrostimulation [19]. Two cases with stage I seminoma showed nodal relapse (Table 3). One case with seminoma showed lymph node relapse at the para-aortic lymph node at the level of left renal vein 10 months after laparoscopic RPLND. Another case with seminoma showed lymph node relapse at the right obturator lymph node 20 months after laparoscopic RPLND. These nodal relapse cases were treated with two courses of standard chemotherapy regimen or right obturatory lymph node dissection after chemotherapy.

TABLE 2. Operative data and complications

Median operating time, minutes (range)	209 (131–372)
Average blood loss, ml (range)	10 (scarce to 260)
Peritoneal penetration	
Initial 14 cases	4
Recent 18 cases	2
Postoperative complications	
Prolonged lymphocele	3
Symptomatic lymphocyst	1
Segmental renal infarction	1
Oral intake on the next day	All

TABLE 3. Pathological and follow-up data

Follow-up time, months (range)	22 (2.7–36)
Micrometastasis	
Clinical stage I	3
Clinical stage IIa	1
Nodal relapse	
Stage I	2
Stage IIa or b	0

Discussion

There are many therapeutic options, such as surveillance, RPLND, radiation, and chemotherapy, for low-stage testicular cancer [1,4,8]. Among these treatments, laparoscopic RPLND has been performed by many urologic surgeons [12–14,20–22]. Laparoscopic RPLND via the transperitoneal approach and via the extraperitoneal approach have been reported. Our laparoscopic RPLND is performed via the entirely extraperitoneal approach in the supine poison. This surgical approach was initially reported by gynecologists for staging cervical cancer [23], and has recently been described by urologists.

The important point of the procedure is that the retroperitoneal space be sufficiently developed prior to the modified template lymphadenectomy. With the blunt dissection of an adequate plane and insufflation of carbon dioxide, the retroperitoneal space was widely and easily extended like a dome. Peritoneal penetration during the developing retroperitoneal space is the most troublesome situation in the operation. Under these circumstances an additional port placement is necessary to retract the peritoneum by fin-type retractor, so the surgeon can perform the subsequent procedure. Once the retroperitoneal working space is developed sufficiently, the technique of the lymph node dissection is carried out in the same manner as open conventional surgery (template dissection technique).

Our procedure can be performed in the supine position and provides the wide dome-like working space, having a peritoneal ceiling without bowel mobilization or manipulation. Under the establishment of a wide pneumoretroperitoneal space, The superior hypogastric plexus below the inferior mesenteric and contralateral or bilateral para-aortic sympathetic nerve can be easily identified and preserved with optical magnification. Although meticulous and bloodless dissection is required of the surgeon, hemorrhage is the most frequently encountered problem in RPLND [24]. Bleeding from small vessels is controlled by clamping bipolar coagulation. In most cases small hemorrhage from the vena cava is controlled by compression of the bleeding point with fine gauze for several minutes. If compression is not efficacious for hemostasis, hemorrhage can be stopped with the help of fibrin glue [14]. If conversion to open surgery is needed, the surgeon can rapidly approach the great vessels by excising the parietal peritoneum after laparotomy via the midline incision.

The technique of extending the retroperitoneal space in the supine position is applicable to various urologic surgeries which are often performed in the flank position [25,26]. When bilateral surgery or consecutive open surgery in the supine position is required, the surgeon does not need to change the position.

In the present study, micrometastasis was found at the radiopositive nodes in two stage I cases who underwent gamma probe-guided RPLND. These radiopositive lymph nodes were easily detected by gamma probe guidance intraoperatively.

The diagnostic and therapeutic accuracy according to sentinel lymph node status may be proved after more extensive experience and follow-up. In the near future, only sentinel node dissection may be a sufficient diagnostic procedure.

In our experience, two stage I cases showed nodal relapse, but the relapse was thought to originate from intraoperative sentinel lymph node detection error and dissection technique error caused by the immature technique of a surgeon with limited experience. In another node relapse case, the relapsed node existed in the right obturator nerve area. Such a case might have another route of lymphatic drainage into the pelvic lymph node, which could not be detected by intratunica albuginea injection of radioactive tracer.

Extraperitoneal laparoscopic RPLND is technically feasible and decreases postoperative morbidity. This technique of developing the retroperitoneal space in the supine position is applicable to various urologic surgeries. The longer follow-up is necessary to determine therapeutic efficacy.

References

1. Spermon JR, Roeleveld TA, Poel HG, Hulsbergen CA, Tenbokkelhunink WW, Vijver M, Witjes JA, Horenblass S (2002) Comparison of surveillance and retroperitoneal lymphnode dissection in stage I nonseminatous germ cell tumors. Urology 59:923–929
2. Recker F, Tsholl R (1993) Monitoring of emission as direct intraoperative control for nerve sparing retroperitoneal lymphadenectomy. J Urol 150:1360–1364
3. Colleselli K, Poisel S, Shchtner W, Bartsch G (1990) Nerve-preserving bilateral retroperitoneal lymphadenectomy: anatomical study and operative approach. J Urol 144:293–298
4. Nicolai N, Pizzicalo G (1995) A surveillance study of clinical stage I nonseminomatous germ cell tumors of the testis. J Urol 154:1045–1049
5. Janetschek G, Hobisch A, Peschel R, Hittmair A, Bartsch G (2000) Laparoscopic retroperitoneal lymph node dissection for clinical stage I nonseminomatous testicular carcinoma: long-term outcome. J Urol 163:1793–1796
6. Suzuki K, Orikasa S, Hoshi S, Yoshikawa K, Imai Y, Aizawa M, Nishimura Y, Okada Y, Ohnuma T, Ogata Y (1998) Surveillance study for clinical I testicular seminomas and nonseminomas germ cell tumors. Int J Urol 5:568–574
7. Duchesne GM, Horwich A, Dearnaley DP, Nicholls J, Jay G, Peckham MJ, Hendry WF (1990) Orchidectomy alone for stage I seminoma of the testis. Cancer 65:1115–1118
8. Hahn EW, Feingold SM, Simpson L, Batata M (1982) Recovery from aspermia induced by low-dose radiation in seminoma patients. Cancer 50:337–340
9. Yeoh E, Horowitz M, Russo A, Muecke T, Robb T, Chatterton B (1995) The effects of abdominal irradiation for seminoma of the testis on gastrointestinal function. J Gastroenterol Hepatol 10:125–130
10. Van Leeuwen FE, Stinggebout AM, Van Den Belt-Dusebout AW, Noyon R, Eliel MR, Van Kerkhoff EH, Delenmarre JF, Somers R (1993) Second cancer risk following testicular cancer: a follow-up study of 1,909 patients. J Clin Oncol 11:2286–2287
11. Rassweiler J, Tsivian A, Kumar AV, Lymberakis C, Schulze M, Seeman O, Frede T (2003) Oncological safety of laparoscopic surgery for urological malignancy: experience with more than 1,000 operations. J Urol 169:2072–2075

12. Bhayani SB, Ong A, Oh WK, Kantoff PW, Kavoussi LR (2003) Laparoscopic retroperitoneal lymph node dissection for clinical stage I nonseminomatous germ cell testicular cancer: a long-term update. Urology 62:324–327
13. Janetschek G, Peschel R, Hobisch A, Bartsch G (2001) Laparoscopic retroperitoneal lymph node dissection. J Endourol 15:449–453
14. Gerber GS, Bissada NK, Hulbert JC, Kavoussi LR, Moore RG, Kantoff PW, Rukstalis DB (1994) Laparoscopic retroperitoneal lymphadenectomy: multi-institutional analysis. J Urol 152:1188–1191
15. Ohyama C, Chiba Y, Yamazaki T, Endoh M, Hoshi S, Arai Y (2002) Lymphatic mapping and gamma probe guided laparoscopic biopsy of sentinel lymph node in patients with clinical stage I testicular tumor. J Urol 168:1390–1395
16. Satoh M, Ito A, Kaiho Y, Nakagawa H, Saito S, Endo M, Ohyama C, Arai Y (2005) Intraoperative radio-guided sentinel lymph node mapping in laparoscopic lymph node dissection for stage I testicular cancer. Cancer: 103:2067–2072
17. Das S (1996) Laparoscopic staging pelvic lymphadenectomy: extraperitoneal approach. Semin Surg Oncol 12:134–138
18. Holtl L, Peschel R, Knapp R, Janetschek G, Steiner H, Hittmair A, Rogatsch H, Bartsch G, Hobisch A (2002) Primary lymphatic metastatic spread in testicular cancer occurs ventral to the lumbar vessels. Urology 59:114–118
19. Kaiho Y, Nakagawa H, Takeuchi A, Ito A, Satoh M, Kurokawa K, Arai Y (2003) Electrostimulation of sympathetic nerve fibers during nerve-sparing laparoscopic retroperitoneal lymph node dissection in testicular tumor. Int J Urol 10:284–286
20. Janetschek G, Hobisch A, Holtl L, Bartsch G (1996) Retroperitoneal lymphadenectomy for clinical stage I nonseminomatous testicular tumor: laparoscopy versus open surgery and impact of learning curve. J Urol 156:89–93
21. LeBlanc E, Caty A, Dargent D, Querleu D, Mazeman E (2001) Extraperitoneal laparoscopic para-aortic lymph node dissection for early-stage nonseminomatous germ cell tumors of the testis with introduction of a nerve sparing technique: description and results. J Urol 165:89–92
22. Hsu TH, Su LM, Ong A (2003) Anterior extraperitoneal approach to laparoscopic retroperitoneal lymph node dissection: a novel technique. J Urol 169:258–260
23. Vasilev SA, McGonigle KF (1996) Extraperitoneal laparoscopic para-aortic lymph node dissection. Gynecol Oncol 61 :315–320
24. Janetschek G (2001) Laparoscopic retroperitoneal lymph node dissection. Urol Clin North Am 28:107–114
25. Gill IS, Clayman RV, Albala DM, Aso Y, Chiu AW, Das S, Donovan JF, Fuchs GJ, Gaur DD, Go H, Gomella LG, Grune MT, Harewood LM, Janetschek G, Knapp PM, McDougall EM, Nakada SY, Preminger GM, Puppo P, Rassweiler JJ, Royce PL, Thomas R, Urban DA Winfield HN (1998) Retroperitoneal and pelvic extraperitoneal laparoscopy: an international perspective. Urology 52:566–571
26. Fugita OE, Jarrett TW, Kavoussi P, Kavoussi LR (2002) Laparoscopic treatment of retroperitoneal fibrosis. J Endourol 16:571–574

Subject Index

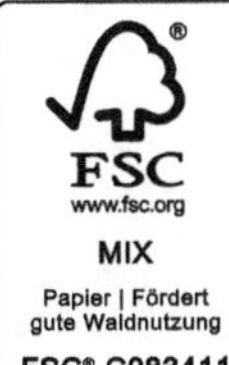

Zeitfracht Medien GmbH
Ferdinand-Jühlke-Straße 7
99095 Erfurt, Deutschland
produktsicherheit@kolibri360.de